The Healthcare Debate

Recent Titles in
Historical Guides to Controversial Issues in America

The Pro-Life/Choice Debate
Mark Y. Herring

Genetic Engineering
Mark Y. Herring

Same-Sex Marriage
Allene Phy-Olsen

Three Strikes Laws
Jennifer E. Walsh

Juvenile Justice
Laura L. Finley

The Welfare Debate
Greg M. Shaw

The Gambling Debate
Richard A. McGowan

Censorship
Mark Paxton

The Torture and Prisoner Abuse Debate
Laura L. Finley

Affirmative Action
John W. Johnson and Robert P. Green, Jr.

Alternative Energy
Brian C. Black and Richard Flarend

The Healthcare Debate

Greg M. Shaw

Historical Guides to Controversial Issues in America

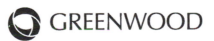 GREENWOOD

AN IMPRINT OF ABC-CLIO, LLC
Santa Barbara, California • Denver, Colorado • Oxford, England

Library of Congress Cataloging-in-Publication Data

Shaw, Greg M.
    The healthcare debate / Greg M. Shaw.
        p. cm. — (Historical guides to controversial issues in America)
    Includes bibliographical references and index.
    ISBN 978-0-313-35666-7 (hard copy : alk. paper) — ISBN 978-0-313-35667-4
    (ebook)
1. Social medicine—United States. 2. Medical care—United States. I. Title.
RA418.3.U6S53   2010
362.1—dc22   2009053669

ISBN: 978-0-313-35666-7
EISBN: 978-0-313-35667-4

14 13 12 11 10   1 2 3 4 5

This book is also available on the World Wide Web as an eBook.
Visit www.abc-clio.com for details.

Greenwood
An Imprint of ABC-CLIO, LLC

ABC-CLIO, LLC
130 Cremona Drive, P.O. Box 1911
Santa Barbara, California 93116-1911

This book is printed on acid-free paper ∞

Manufactured in the United States of America

Contents

List of Tables and Figures

TABLES

FIGURES

Preface

Writing a book about the debates surrounding healthcare policy reminds one, over and over again, of just how little the arguments actually have to do with health. Instead, the disputes about how to provide quality coverage to a greater portion of the population at affordable prices have strongly tended to focus on professional autonomy for health providers, notions of appropriate roles for government, and money, though not necessarily in that order.

This book traces the long-running debate over health care in an effort to help those who know a little about it to learn more, and to help those who know more to put their perspectives in a historical context. The chapters that follow describe both the changes and the continuities in the expert and general public discourses about how the medical profession has struggled to define itself, how government actors have at times supported and at other moments opposed a greater public-sector role in healthcare financing, and how interest groups and the public have contested matters of medical cost, quality, and access since the early 1800s.

One of the challenges of writing a short book on health care is the matter of scope. The themes range far and wide over a rapidly evolving landscape of public health issues; changing roles for government in financing and monitoring health outcomes; the rise of a massive insurance industry; labor market practices, including many recent developments in employer-employee relations in an age of nearly untenable retirement health benefit plans; technology-driven medical inflation; the changing character of the American Medical Association (AMA)—and the list goes on. In an effort to make this history of the debate over health care in America manageable, I have focused it rather sharply on government involvement in public health, and healthcare financing and delivery. This lens provides useful perspectives not only on how Americans think about and have thought about the meaning of *public* in public health but also on the highly important implications of the evolving understanding of basic health care as a right of citizenship.

Americans have for a very long time professed to resist government insinuation into the doctor-patient relationship. At the same time they have gradually availed themselves of greater government roles, in everything from mandatory vaccinations that helped stamp out the great plagues of the nineteenth century to the screening of new pharmaceuticals, medical service financing for tens of millions of retirees and people with modest incomes, and monitoring the corporate practices of health maintenance organizations. One might imagine a tension between the profession of a laissez-faire approach to medicine, as a matter of symbols and language, and the very real fact of deep and wide government involvement, involvement that might be poorly understood but is cherished all the same. An anecdote from the 1990s illustrates this point. A woman attending a town hall meeting where President Clinton's reform plan was being discussed finally reached the end of her patience with all the talk of government involvement in medicine. She stood up and proclaimed, with a bit of unintended irony borne of ignorance, "Next thing you know, the government will want to take over Medicare!"[1]

Like it or not, government involvement in healthcare delivery and financing appears to be here to stay. But that does not end the debate over just how those programs should work, how effectively they do work, or which among the wide range of as-yet-untried options should be employed. Given the steeply rising cost of health care to the nation, 7 percent of our gross national product in 1970, just over 16 percent in 2008, and projected to exceed 30 percent by the year 2030, these issues will only grow in importance. As evolving medical technology continues to escalate costs, employers increasingly face daunting questions of how to finance benefits for their workers. Further, as baby boomers continue to enter retirement, debates over health care have assumed a place of importance alongside the other first-tier issues facing the nation. This book attempts to situate the current healthcare discourse in a historic context to help readers make sense of what is likely to remain a dominant issue for the current generation and well into the foreseeable future.

Despite the many discouraging aspects of the state of health and healthcare programs in the United States, this project has been a joy on which to work. Many people along the way deserve thanks. Sandy Towers at Greenwood/ABC-CLIO has been a pleasure to work with in her unfailing helpfulness and good humor. Several current and former students at Illinois Wesleyan University provided excellent research assistance, including Nate Erickson, Christine Gibbs, Ryan Lambert, Scott Miller, Bobby Porter, Julie Regenbogen, Chelsea Schafer, Erin Strauts, Amy Uden, and Emily Vock. Thanks to Sarah Keister for her helpful comments on early versions of the manuscript. Conversations with Roger Hunt, Bill DeLong, and Penny Cermak at Advocate BroMenn Medical Center helped me see things I never would have on my own. Lauren Dodge and Tony Heaton at Illinois Wesleyan University kindly offered their fine librarianship, as did the library staff at the University of Illinois at Urbana-Champaign and at Rush University Medical Center in Chicago. Financial support from Illinois Wesleyan facilitated several parts of this project, including travel and research materials. I am grateful to my children, Ian and Fiona, for their patience during what has been a busy time. To the two people to whom this book is dedicated I give heartfelt thanks. Mollie Ward deserves recognition for all she gave in the way of support and insights into the world of health care, for patiently reading manuscript drafts, and much more. Bob Shapiro at Columbia University also has my deep gratitude for all he has taught me throughout the years. Of course, any remaining errors in the text are my own.

NOTE

1. Peterson 1995, p. 427.

Introduction: Why No National Health Insurance in America?

The United States is the world's only industrialized democracy without a national health insurance program. How exceptional that fact makes the United States is not open to much debate. Several related questions, on the other hand, lend themselves to considerable argument: why this is so, whether government should do something about it, and if so, just what might be done. On the first question, several schools of thought have contended over the past half century or so without much resulting consensus. About as close as policy analysts have come to resolving this is to boil down the possible answers mainly to two. The first assumes that the American lack of national health insurance is a function of attitudes or interests that stand opposed to activist government in general or to government involvement in the healthcare sector in particular.[1] A variant strand of this argument posits that Americans want national health insurance but are perpetually ambivalent about how to design it, thus they cannot find a concrete way to act on their desire. Lastly, some argue that most Americans want national health insurance but that powerful organized interests stand in the way of majority public opinion getting what it wants. These are the attitudinal explanations.

The second school of thought looks to our political institutions and sees there an array of pitfalls that somehow always manage to trip up well-intentioned policy reformers, advocates who may even enjoy majority public support, usually by way of providing interest groups—health insurance companies, professional medical associations, antitax groups, and the like—lots of opportunities to waylay otherwise smart reforms while on their very circuitous path to becoming law. Because of the necessity to assemble supermajorities in many political venues at once, policy making in a context of separated institutions that share power, such as ours, faces multiple stop-look-listen-and-reconsider signs. Political scientists refer to this sort of thing as a process marked by multiple veto points. We will call this the institutional explanation. In the interest of truth in advertising, be warned: this book won't settle this debate. But it will give readers a lot to think about as they wrestle with these possible explanations.[2]

Answers to the second question, whether government should do something about it, usually turn on the political ideology of the person being asked, his or her beliefs about health care as a basic right of citizenship (sort of like K-12 education), whether one has a financial stake in the current system of healthcare financing and delivery, and whether government versus private-market mechanisms are most appropriate to extend healthcare access across more of the population than is covered now. Fairly few people today argue that we need less health care or less good quality medical care in America. But the question of whether it is the role of government to provide coverage quickly runs into a deep divide between conservatives' market sensibilities and liberals' eagerness to see government as a workable solution. As government-sponsored health programs have expanded incrementally—chiefly, under Medicare and Medicaid—more Americans have grown accustomed to public-sector involvement in healthcare financing. This evolution has not, however, altogether convinced the political Right, or the AMA, or the insurance industry, that more of the same would be a good thing. The chapters that follow trace how the debate over health care in the United States has reflected these core disagreements over time and how the evolution of government and healthcare delivery, including the rise of professional medicine in the mid-1800s, the birth of the modern insurance industry in the second quarter of the twentieth century, and more recent trials of managed care have changed how we tend to think about government's role in health.

The third theme, what Americans might do to address the crippling costs of medical services, is the subject of the book's final chapter. Several possible reforms are discussed, some of which were actively under debate at the time this book went to press. This discussion also helps to knit together the continuities and the changes in the healthcare debate over the past century and a half. This book is not a how-to guide for healthcare reformers but rather strives to integrate historical lessons with contemporary debates.

As readers will have surmised, healthcare provision is hard to think about for several reasons. First, the goals of various reform movements have changed through time, from expansion of public expenditures in the early twentieth century, to attempts at greater equity of coverage through redistribution in the 1960s, to efforts to stop or slow growth, at least in terms of cost, in the late twentieth century.[3] As the edifice under construction has changed, so too have the strategies of the architects. Simply put, the kinds of arguments that made sense in the late nineteenth or early twentieth centuries make a lot less sense now. Further, Americans have moved toward but have not quite arrived at a consensus that some level of basic medical care ought to be a right of citizenship. Until this issue is settled, arguments about whether health care works like other economic markets will continue as obstacles to public provision of these services. The problem of Americans as ideologically conservative but programmatically liberal also plagues the business of trying to fit proposed policies to public preferences. So long as a broad swath of the public expresses distaste for proposed big-government fixes to societal problems in the abstract while at the same time it defends particular programs from which it benefits in tangible ways, having a coherent conversation about the costs and consequences of a national health program will prove very difficult.

One of the more important arguments that has played a central role since the rise of health insurance in the 1930s is that medical service allocation should be treated like any other economic market. Goods and services in most markets are consumed in line with consumers' preferences, tastes, and ability to pay. Insurance or public aid, absent aggressive cost-sharing provisions (such as large co-payments), so goes this argument developed beginning in the 1960s, creates a moral hazard, reducing the cost of those services to the consumer, creating a prisoner's dilemma in which no consumer sees the wisdom of reducing his or her consumption even though such reductions would make everyone better off.[4] This is the starting point for the contemporary consumer-driven healthcare movement carried on by various conservative and libertarian advocates. The problem, in the view of a very broad range of analysts who think differently about these matters, is that medical service consumption is characterized by a poor fit between preferences and consumption. Presumably, no one learns of a new type of intestinal surgical procedure and, independent of the physical need for it, decides to purchase one.[5] In modern times, only at a limited margin do individuals increase or decrease their consumption of medical services based on their preference or ability to pay. Some evidence indicates that cost does affect consumption, though this evidence applies best to those above a certain minimum threshold and does not speak very well to the sick poor.[6] Uninsured people who are critically ill or injured go to emergency rooms, and the resulting costs (amounting to approximately $35 billion in uncompensated care in 2001) are shifted to those of us who are insured.[7] Wealthy people do not routinely buy fancier health care to the same extent they buy fancier cars or clothes. Specifically, demand for services is not driven directly by patients but by the vicissitudes of one's physical health and by doctors as they decide what treatments to apply, decisions that rarely involve doctors explaining to patients what one course of treatment as opposed to another might cost. The problem on this latter point, of course, is that business relationships develop between doctors and medical goods vendors (such as drug companies that give doctors incentives to prescribe their medicines) that disempower patients and drive up costs through incestuous means.[8] The upshot is that there are very few truly informed buyers in health care, if by such people we are talking about patients.

The bottom line is that health care is not like other efficient economic markets.[9] In this crucial sense, healthcare purchasing differs from behavior regarding most other consumer goods and makes market-based solutions to healthcare coverage deeply problematic, since the relationship between what one pays for insurance and what one gets in return is only very loosely related, and that only through either the steepness of one's co-payments or the size and demographic composition of the insurance pool one buys into. Given this, it is probably impossible to design an economically efficient insurance-based financing system that gives individual rewards directly in line with consumer choices. Shifting to a purely out-of-pocket payment system would move in a direction that honors the market somewhat more, but only somewhat, and along the way it would run afoul of the multibillion dollar-a-year insurance industry and would completely dismiss any notion of social insurance, a notion that has become central to much of contemporary American life.

So we are left with a debate over health care that perhaps most usefully aims to sort out just what we mean by citizenship and the extent to which healthcare access should be conceived of as a fundamental right. As healthcare policy expert Deborah Stone has written, "the politics of health insurance can only be understood as a struggle over the meaning of sickness and whether it should be a condition that automatically generates mutual assistance."[10] Our skepticism should be triggered when anyone tells us that we must interpret a problem in a given way, but Stone's perspective is indeed a compelling one. If the alternative to thinking in terms of a health politics of mutual aid is one of a healthcare politics of actuarial fairness, that is, allowing people to avoid others' risks, then large-scale, general-admission insurance pools should be rejected along with any attempt to limit the scrutiny of underwriters as they poke and prod into our individual health backgrounds and genetic makeup. Obviously, both these ideas run counter to current norms. This in turn may steer us around to conclude that we are all in this together, in which case national health insurance comes to make a lot more sense than its critics have historically admitted. That, however, is up to Americans to decide.

THE PLAN OF THE BOOK

Chapter 1 presents a brief history of some of the more important developments in American medicine from the 1700s through the first decade of the twentieth century. Understanding the broad outlines of the debates over what constituted mainstream medicine, as opposed to alternative healing arts, is interesting in itself but is also useful in illustrating how early steps to govern medicine were halting at best and reflected a still-robust resistance to perceived interference in the doctor-patient relationship and financially-based resentment to government intrusion into physicians' ability to be autonomous business entrepreneurs. The evolution of modern medicine and the medical industry offers interesting insights, and this chapter uses those to illustrate why the politics of health care during the Progressive Era unfolded as it did.

When the Progressive reforms of the early twentieth century swept into federal law workers' compensation, unemployment insurance, and finally the Social Security Act of 1935, they did not include medical insurance, despite vigorous attempts by proponents of national plans to do so. This failure of Progressive Era and later New Deal advocates to enact some sort of national health program is the topic of Chapter 2, spanning the 1910s through 1950. The resulting drift through the 1950s into the 1960s, discussed in Chapter 3, was a period seemingly without much direction for either health reformers or their opposition. This somewhat paradoxical time, during which liberal advocates settled for tiny steps forward—principally federal grants for hospital construction and a small reimbursement program to pay medical expenses for poor people—was also a time of gradual lessening of resistance to government involvement in health from the AMA and its allies. Turning the tide decisively at the end of this period and opening the door for the creation of Medicare and Medicaid in 1965 were the election of John Kennedy in 1960 and the Democrats' later victories in the elections of 1964. The story of the creation of these two pillars of America's welfare state is discussed in Chapter 4.

Following the significant steps forward for public health care advocates embodied by Medicare and Medicaid, these two programs gradually expanded through the 1970s and 1980s, but so did healthcare costs more generally. These developments—including the inauguration of government oversight of modern health maintenance organizations, a short-lived effort to cover catastrophic illnesses under Medicare (itself a catastrophic political failure), and rates of medical inflation combined with incremental expansions to Medicaid—gradually refocused the nation's attention on this issue, as discussed in Chapter 5. The increasingly aggressive bite that medical expenses came to take out of both public and private budgets resulted in the issue that once more became a first-tier campaign theme for politicians in the early 1990s. The bold but unsuccessful plan for government-managed competition offered by Bill and Hillary Clinton, described in Chapter 6, taught healthcare reformers a hard lesson about the difficulty of overcoming both the attitudinal and institutional obstacles to effecting significant change to a sector that accounts for one-seventh of the nation's economy. In the years that immediately followed, perhaps ironically, the failure of government-shepherded managed care gave way to market-based efforts at managed care, changes that spurred deep resentments among medical providers and consumers alike. The rise and fall of health maintenance organizations and other developments from the late 1990s to the present are discussed in Chapter 7.

Chapter 8 reviews some lessons learned over the past century and a half to put the current push for healthcare reform by the Obama administration in context. In the end, popular and interest group resistance to government interventions in the market has limited the political power of calls for sweeping reforms that might provide universal access even to basic health services. When those calls have been made, institutional fragmentation has played a major part in their frustration. To the extent this latter issue blocks popular reform efforts, Americans, regardless of their attitudes toward the idea of health care as a basic right of citizenship, will likely progress in changed policy only in fits and starts for as far as the eye can see.

NOTES

1. See Jacobs 1993b.
2. See Steinmo and Watts 1995 for a thoughtful discussion of these explanations.
3. See Starr 1982, pp. 337–338, for discussion of this point.
4. See Pauly 1968.
5. For the early statement of this insight, see Arrow 1963. For a more recent one, see Stone 1993.
6. See Newhouse 1993.
7. Coombs 2005, p. 263.
8. See Relman 2007, chapter 1 for discussion.
9. Some disagree with this statement. See Epstein 1997 for one example.
10. Stone 1993, p. 290.

1

Setting the Stage: Uncertainty in Early Medicine and Government Roles

Government efforts to advance public health in the United States over the first century of the republic confronted multiple obstacles, including poor knowledge about the causes and treatments of diseases, deep divisions among healers regarding best practices, an underdeveloped vision of the state as a provider or facilitator of medical care, shortages of formally trained care givers, poverty, and problems with public infrastructure ranging from few clinics and hospitals to open sewers and a lack of clean drinking water, and other factors. Practices that could fairly be called modern medicine did not prevail in America until the end of the nineteenth century, and even then wide-ranging debates ensued regarding medical education and practice and the appropriate role of the federal and state governments in making available even basic health care to the mass public. Some of the current debates over health in the United States trace their roots to those of the early nineteenth century. Other threads in the debate grew out of more recent developments, such as the matter of formal medical school curricula and political goals that Progressive Era health insurance advocates were not permitted to accomplish. The entanglement of public and private concerns that marked health care throughout the first century of the republic raised themes and disagreements that echoed forward through time, some to the present day. In order to appreciate more fully how intractable some of the lines of the healthcare debate are, it is useful to review a bit of history. This chapter undertakes that task.

Because of the small population and the extensive wilderness, the North American continent seemed rather hygienic to most early European immigrants who, in the case of those coming from settled areas, would have suffered through the filth and periodic epidemics that plagued the crowded cities of Europe. In time, however, not only would European settlers experience their own infectious epidemics—typhoid, malaria, yellow fever, and cholera were among the more common illnesses—but also they would share their deadly germs, sometimes accidentally and sometimes intentionally, with the indigenous people, particularly small pox, in many cases wiping out entire Native American communities.[1] Throughout the late 1600s and early 1700s, with the growth of larger cities and towns, the colonists began to confront serious epidemics and to realize the need to regulate public health somewhat more aggressively than they had in the earliest years of settlement. In 1666 Boston appointed its first scavenger, a public employee who was responsible for removing the carcasses of dead animals found around the city. In time this practice spread.[2]

From the early eighteenth century forward, concerns about public health preoccupied government officials, particularly in the growing urban centers of the East. As a practical matter, cities and towns were severely limited in what they could do, given their scarce resources and the rather ad hoc ways in which early cities grew. Zoning codes were uncommon until the late 1800s, so dirty industrial sites could be located in proximity to residential areas, and open sewer systems were common well into the nineteenth century, providing a breeding ground for pestilence. Prior to the development of the first vaccines in the early 1700s, quarantines were a primary tool for combating the spread of infectious diseases, but they were only marginally effective, given the difficulty of their enforcement by weak governments. By the 1720s, concern over small pox epidemics ran sufficiently high that several states passed mandatory quarantine laws, including Rhode Island's stipulation that anyone caught concealing a case of the disease would be put to death "without benefit of clergy."[3] Fears of disease-bearing immigrants prompted other eastern cities and states to consider quarantine laws as well. By the mid-1740s, quarantine of both Europeans and African slaves in the local "pest house" became common practice.[4] These laws were a patchwork, however, enforced mainly by town and city governments in the North and primarily by state governments in the South. Quarantines were used in 1832 in the major cities of the eastern United States to try to ward off cholera, which was known to have afflicted England that spring. New Yorkers had particular reason to be concerned, as the city's sanitation was abysmal, owing in no small part to the thousands of swine that roamed the streets at will in the early 1830s.[5] New York's Board of Health had experienced approximately a dozen large-scale epidemics prior to the 1832 outbreak of cholera, and it assumed control of sanitation, slum clearance, and hospital and welfare functions during the 1832 epidemic. This is not to say that the city government responded with particular efficiency. Politically well-connected saloon keepers remained free to ply their trade as usual throughout the 1832 epidemic.[6]

Significantly incomplete records at both federal and state levels regarding illness rates prior to the end of the nineteenth century make good estimates of the scope of epidemics hard to come by, though tens of thousands died in the cholera outbreaks of the 1830s, 1840s, and 1860s. The U.S. Census Bureau did not include questions about health, such as tracking the number of blind people, until 1830, and states made little progress even in the relatively straightforward matter of counting births and deaths in a systematic way prior to 1900.[7] It is, however, clearer that weak governments combined with poverty and poor medical knowledge made combating epidemics a grave challenge for public health officials in early America.

EARLY MEDICAL KNOWLEDGE

A significant obstacle to early efforts toward public health, and medical practice more generally, was the poor state of knowledge regarding the causes of disease and effective medical strategies to combat them. Systematic medical knowledge expanded in Europe throughout the 1700s but only very slowly made its way to the American colonies. Although the first American medical society was formed in Boston in 1735 and another in New York in 1749, the flow of medical knowledge across the Atlantic proceeded only gradually. By the mid-1700s enough knowledge had accumulated to foster a contentious divide between what were called regular physicians and other practitioners, who, despite their widely varying approaches, were often lumped together under the label of eclectics or seculars. The latter included homeopaths, osteopaths, chiropractors, suggestive therapists, magnetic healers, spondylotherapaths, water therapists, primitive psychotherapists, naprapaths, mechnotherapaths, electrotherapaths, naturopaths, and religious healers, among others.[8] A wide variety of schools of thought regarding healing flourished in the United States during the first half of the nineteenth century. Samuel Thompson patented his first botanical mixtures in 1813 as a response to the common use—overuse, he believed—of antimony, mercury, and purgatives.[9] Homeopathy arrived from France in the mid-1820s, and the American Institute of Homeopathy was founded in 1844. Andrew Still instituted the practice of osteopathy in 1874 and founded the American School of Osteopathy in 1892. Daniel Palmer founded the chiropractic movement in 1895 in Davenport, Iowa. Chiropractors' efforts to win recognition would eventually lead them to gain licensure in all 50 states by the late twentieth century, though chiropractics would be referred to as "quacks" by the American Medical Association (AMA) until they successfully sued that organization in 1983 for restraint of trade.[10]

Christian Science was launched with the publication of *Science and Health* in 1875. The American Electro-Therapeutic Association was founded in 1891.[11]

Mainstream medicine scorned the eclectics, but in the early 1800s America proved fertile ground for alternative practitioners. Obtaining a conventional medical education was, in fact, something of a challenge, often involving travel to Europe.[12] Prior to 1800, only five regular medical schools operated in the United States, all founded between 1764 and 1798.[13] Consequently, until the beginning of the twentieth century American medical practice resided in low esteem among European physicians. Many physicians in the early 1800s who considered themselves conventional nonetheless followed some curious detours, including some of dubious efficacy and others that were outright dangerous. Phrenology, which held some sway during the early 1800s, involved measuring skulls in order to correlate their shapes and sizes with various personality types and medical disorders. Beyond this, some of the more heroic approaches employed bleeding, blistering, and purging. A lingering belief in the body's four humors—blood, black and yellow bile, and phlegm—led practitioners to pursue bloodletting and sweat regimens in order to restore patients' physiological equilibrium. George Washington was likely a famous casualty of this sort of treatment—along with an unhealthy dose of mercury chloride in his case, another common remedy of the period—that flourished in early America.

In time, the humor theory of disease gave way to environmental explanations for illness, specifically the miasmatic theory, which dominated medical thinking until late in the nineteenth century. This view held that an invisible but dangerous substance emanated from the earth and infected its victims. Miasmatic explanations found support in the observation that malaria outbreaks always began in neighborhoods nearest the water. Only later did the presence of infected mosquitoes occur to malaria investigators.[14] Environmental explanations for disease were slow to force out the humor school of thought. Not until the 1840s did blood-letting experience moderation by mainstream practitioners.[15] Defining the mainstream required a significant passage of time. The battles began by the mid-1700s. In 1757 the American historian William Smith noted, "Few physicians among us are eminent for their skill. Quacks abound like locusts in Egypt."[16] In 1800, Dr. John Sterns, founder of the New York State Medical Society, complained that "with a few, honorable exceptions . . . practitioners [of medicine] were ignorant, degraded and contemptible."[17] Precisely these sorts of complaints led to the formation of the AMA in 1847.

Early medicine not only appeared grim in the eyes of many contemporary observers, but the records that exist show how ineffective it was. Looking at one salient indicator of health, infant mortality, shows how little the practice of medicine improved the lives of early Americans. In the mid-eighteenth century infant mortality rates stood between 150 and 200 deaths per 1,000 live births, somewhat higher in rural areas than in urban ones, probably due to less access to medical care and the relative unavailability of midwives. (Compare this rate to the contemporary U.S. rate of just over 6.2 deaths per 1,000 live births.[18]) Rates of infant mortality among southern slaves were approximately twice the rates among southern whites.[19] Beyond infections, perhaps tuberculosis primary among them, child birth was a highly risky activity for eighteenth-century women, and poorer ones stood substantially greater risk of death in child labor than wealthier ones.[20]

A few early discoveries gradually advanced medical progress. One of the more significant medical breakthroughs was the emergence of vaccines in the early 1700s. A live vaccine strategy for small pox was articulated as early as the 1710s in a British medical journal. By the 1770s small pox inoculations were common.[21] Safer and more effective cow pox vaccines were developed in the 1790s, so that by the early nineteenth century, small pox ceased being a leading cause of death among infants.[22] Massachusetts adopted a law in the early 1800s that required communities to undertake small pox vaccination campaigns, though because the law had no enforcement mechanism, it fell far short of its potential despite the commonwealth's willingness to pay for the program. Realizing the public benefit, the city of New Orleans paid for small pox vaccines for the poor in 1817. State authority came to play further on this issue when some traditional-minded doctors clung to the earlier, more dangerous vaccines, which led some states to outlaw their use, such as New York's legislation against them in 1816. Maryland did so as late as 1850.[23]

GOVERNMENT INVOLVEMENT IN PUBLIC HEALTH AND MEDICINE

President Franklin Pierce's 1854 veto of a bill to fund mental health facilities, a measure championed by the noted social activist Dorothea Dix, is often cited by scholars as emblematic of the antebellum embrace of a minimalist federal government. Pierce argued that he saw no constitutional provision for such an exercise of congressional power.[24] That veto, while important, should not be understood as widely held objection to all government involvement in public health. From the beginning of the 1700s and more commonly from the 1830s forward, communities across the country provided asylums for the mentally and chronically ill along with the poor. Care for the sick in asylums or poorhouses was typically provided by a physician whom the town engaged on a lowest-bidder basis; that is, the doctor willing to perform the work for the least amount typically won the contract.[25] Community hospitals were built from the early 1700s.[26] The vast majority of these early hospitals were privately operated on a nonprofit basis—most of them Episcopalian by affiliation—and provided care mainly for the poor, as families of means typically placed greater trust in home-based physician care. These facilities, prominently among them Massachusetts General, New York's St. Luke's, and Pennsylvania Hospital, offered physicians places to often practice pro bono medicine as part of their cultivation of community standing. By the early 1870s there were some 150 such community hospitals around the country.[27] In addition to these sectarian hospitals, by the 1850s most larger towns and cities operated poorhouses or asylums for the chronically ill, along with the poor. Part of the impetus for these government efforts turned on a humanitarian impulse, although they were also motivated by a desire to protect citizens from the unpredictability of the mentally ill who would otherwise live among them.[28] As urbanization advanced throughout the first quarter of the nineteenth century, large-scale public health problems emerged with increasing frequency in larger cities and towns.[29] The social and economic dislocation of this era not only aggravated the plight of poor workers who struggled to make ends meet but also frustrated the public boards of health, which tended to be weakly organized and often ineffective, with the strong exception during the second quarter of the nineteenth century being that of Boston. In the 1860s New York formed a highly capable city health department, and Chicago did the same in 1867 in response to anxiety surrounding the cholera outbreak in 1865.[30]

Amid these efforts to make government an active player in advancing public health resided an uncertainty about how to navigate the deepening divide between various sects of medical practitioners. During much of the first half of the 1800s a widely held distrust of medical professionals persisted, which led to most of the early boards of health, dating back to the late 1700s, being controlled by laypeople.[31] Acrimony within the medical community over the causes of disease imparted a sense that a health board consisting entirely of physicians would prove internally divisive, thus ineffective.[32] By accumulating some objective successes, regular physicians during the mid- to late 1800s gained more credibility, which, in turn, led governments to grant them more prominent roles when designing public health measures. Consequently, public health measures tended to become more concerted.

Tuberculosis was the first disease that garnered significant government action to fight, and it offers a standout example of aggressive government action on health. Through the late 1800s tuberculosis was a primary cause of death in the United States. However, thanks to Trudeau's successful development of a sanatorium treatment for the disease in the 1870s, tax-supported institutions developed quite rapidly to address it. Government payment for tuberculosis treatment made so much sense that even by the 1870s the

imperative to isolate contagious patients was such that most large cities operated dedicated hospitals on their outskirts in order to prevent the spread of
the disease.[33] Because the treatment of tuberculosis was so expensive, it was
beyond the reach of most people to pay for it. Government action to fight
tuberculosis, along with cholera and typhoid, from the middle of the nineteenth century onward, provided a rational basis for increased government
involvement, which took the form of robust state or city boards of public
health. Federal involvement was a different matter, however. In the late
1870s when legislation proposed that the creation of a strong federal public
health agency failed, it became evident that Congress lacked the will to enter
this area that had traditionally been left to state or local control. When in
1879 Congress finally created a National Board of Health, it was a weak body
and was made responsible mainly to monitor quarantines.[34]

Beyond the controversy surrounding the government involvement in quarantines and initial efforts at funding public health measures, a more contentious
early aspect of government involvement in medicine surrounded the matter of
physician licensure. The first of these efforts began in 1760 in New York. Twelve
years later New Jersey enacted a licensure law under which a person wishing to
practice medicine was first to be examined by "any two of the judges of the
Supreme Court."[35] A second wave of licensure laws progressed through the first
quarter of the nineteenth century, and by the 1830s, 13 states had licensing procedures. However, these efforts at control soon collided in America with the
arrival of various eclectic practices and the spirit of Jacksonian democracy and
its notions of antielitism more generally. On the latter point, the growing sense
that government regulation constituted a wading into matters of class fostered
the view that licensing requirements were little more than barriers to entry
into the medical market.[36] On the former point, the arrival of homeopathy in
the 1820s was accompanied by the spread of Thomsonian practices, named
for Samuel Thomas, a practitioner whose treatments were based on an understanding of the body's humors and involved various vegetable treatments, sweat-
ing regimens, and encouraging patients to become their own doctors.
Thomsonianism gained a considerable following through the 1820s and
1830s.[37] The result of this practice and the spread of other eclectic schools of
thought was that over the next decade 11 states repealed their licensing laws
due to pressure from various practitioners who wanted freedom to apply their
healing crafts as they saw fit. State officials were reluctant to arbitrate the increasingly strident arguments between sects. Following this, progress on state licensure provisions would essentially stall until after the Civil War. Beginning in
the 1870s, with progress in medical science, licensure legislation resumed.[38]

Where licensing did occur, there arose the question of what standards to
apply in qualifying practitioners. Debates throughout the early 1800s had

turned on whether an MD degree should be required or instead merely the satisfaction of a medical society exam. At the time, most American doctors did not hold MD degrees. As evidence of the fractured state of the medical discipline, both standards were used across states during this first attempt at licensure. For their part, medical schools argued that their programs were of sufficiently high caliber that no further qualification of their graduates should be required. Further, state legislators were loath to wade into the internecine warfare raging between eclectic and regular schools. Their predisposition was to allow patients to judge for themselves the qualifications of practitioners. Eclectics charged that licensure was nothing more than an attempt by more orthodox physicians to further their own financial monopoly, a claim rejected by the regulars.[39]

THE FOUNDING OF THE AMERICAN MEDICAL ASSOCIATION AND EARLY MEDICAL EDUCATION

As a response to the struggle over medical practices and qualifications, a group of regular physicians came together to form the AMA in 1847. Its constitution stated the organization's purpose was "to promote the science and art of medicine and the betterment of public health."[40] At its 1855 conference the AMA explicitly took a stand against homeopaths in an effort to root out what many regular physicians saw as essentially snake oil salesmen.[41] These early efforts by the AMA were not particularly effective, in as much as it was working against a general public that was not widely convinced of a best school of medical thought and with a group of physicians among whom there persisted significant dissent regarding best practices. Competing medical associations sprang up as counterforces to the AMA, including the Physio-Medical Physicians and Surgeons in 1883, the American Association of Physicians and Surgeons in 1894, and the American Medical Union in 1899. The AMU came together, in their words, in order to "secure the repeal of all medical statues based on the principles of despotic paternalism."[42] Clearly, they chafed at the attempted hegemony of the AMA.

A major challenge facing the regular physicians was their disagreement on matters of medical technique. But this was only a part of the problem. Another aspect of the resistance was financial and had to do with standards for medical education and the autonomy of schools to determine their own curriculum. While the first American medical schools were created in the 1760s as parts of larger universities, by about 1815 small, independent schools appeared, often operated as proprietary businesses of the faculty. Tuition was a significant income source for the instructors, who in turn faced a keen financial incentive to ensure that students graduated and were able to parlay their diplomas into viability in the labor market. Hence, the idea of a licensure exam beyond graduation stood as a threat to the livelihood of these proprietary schools.[43] The profitability of medical schools led to the more than doubling in their numbers between 1830 and 1845. Regular practitioners saw this trend as a watering down of the curriculum compared to schools that relied on a didactic model of lectures, laboratory work, and clinical rotations. This resentment led Dr. Nathan Davis to introduce a resolution at a meeting of the New York State Medical Society in 1845 to call a gathering that would lead to the creation of the AMA.[44] At the first meeting of the AMA a committee on medical education was formed to study the quality of medical school curricula. This inquiry began with the premise that, according to what is essentially the AMA-authorized history of the AMA, from the very outset "the committee had already decided that there were too many doctors in the United States, the proportion being five times as great as France." The committee members voiced concern that "the oversupply of doctors was largely responsible for the rise of quackery and charlatanism," but instead of focusing purely on quality, it urged a curtailing of the number of schools, suggesting that the regular physicians were as concerned about the financial competition as they were about the rigor of instruction.[45] Certainly by this time, doctors, whether part of the AMA, were concerned with a glut of practitioners in the market and about depressed wages.

WOMEN IN MEDICINE

Prior to their entry into the formal ranks of university-trained physicians, women had worked as midwives and healers of various types for generations. Elizabeth Blackwell, the first American woman to earn a medical degree, did so from Geneva Medical College in New York in 1849. Her entry into the profession along with that of many other women generated considerable consternation from many male doctors throughout the second half of the nineteenth century. When the Woman's Medical College in Philadelphia was founded in 1850, a development that reflected the feminist social movement of the time, most physicians "condemned the program in violent terms" due to the threat it posed to their own prestige.[46] For male doctors unwelcoming of the trend—and that probably constituted most male doctors of the time—the threat must have seemed to be closing in around them throughout the 1850s and 1860s, as several coed or purely women's medical colleges opened their doors during that period. Central Medical College, an eclectic school in Syracuse, New York, produced its first female graduates in 1850.[47] A pair of Boston-based private schools also opened during this time, one in 1848 and the other in 1862.[48] Editorials in the *Boston Medical and Surgical Journal* in 1853 sought to bring the "unsettled question" of women in medicine into the open.[49] Male physicians tended to argue that women, by their supposed delicate nature, could not possibly excel at medicine because of their purported inability to cope with the stresses and the grizzly side of the practice, such as dissection and amputations. As John Ware, one male opponent of women physicians, noted, medical instruction with its "ghastly" aspects of "blood and agony" would spoil women by toughening their gentle nature.[50]

Some male physicians appeared to want to have it both ways in their arguments for excluding women from the profession, claiming that women were endowed with well-developed gifts for nursing and that, in many cases, they possessed a moral superiority to men, but that these abilities still did not suit them to be doctors.[51] Interestingly, many women physicians fought back not by contesting the separate spheres idea but rather by explicitly claiming women's natural healing powers as imparted to them through their maternal function. Even the pioneering Elizabeth Blackwell later wrote that women made better healers because they were morally superior to men owing to their "spiritual power of maternity."[52] Arguments against women in medicine also touched on the physiological aspects, asserting that menstruation, still a poorly understood function in the 1860s and 1870s, weakened women, rendering them unable to be relied upon to respond to patients' medical emergencies.[53] Other skeptics adopted an approach that was more blatantly dismissive yet, arguing, as did Dr. Alfred Stillé at the AMA's 1871 convention, that no woman rightly "assumes the first place" in any profession, not even those typically thought of as female professions such as cooking and art. Stillé claimed that the "ignorance, the inexactness, the untrustworthiness, the unbusinesslike ways of women, are appalling" and that women "usually display a strange ignorance of the logic of reason, and a profound contempt for the logic of facts."[54] The seating of Sarah Hackett Stevenson as a member of the Illinois delegation of the AMA in 1876, the first woman to gain admission to the Association's convention, must have provided a moment of historical gravity for all concerned.[55]

One other part of the argument against women in the profession had to do with economics. Throughout the second half of the nineteenth century, organized medicine generated a steady stream of complaints about doctors' poor salaries and how the field was crowded, in the sheer numbers of not only with regular physicians but also with quacks and, increasingly, women, who tended to be placed into the same category with the irregulars. The *Boston Medical and Surgical Journal* complained in 1884 that with more medical schools turning out more new doctors, each year saw an intrusion of "swarms of young men and young women" into an already crowded field. Similarly, an editorial in the *Journal of the American Medical Association* opined in 1898, "Never was the outlook so gloomy, the profession is overcrowded to the starving point."[56]

While certainly inventive, these varied arguments carried the day regarding admission of women to major medical schools until the early 1890s. Not until then did any major medical school accept women. Instead they had to settle for apprenticeships, courses of study at second-tier schools, or study in Europe. The expansion of the land-grant and other state schools in the late nineteenth century, with universities obliged to coed admissions under the terms of their charters, meant that by 1893, 37 of the 105 regular medical schools in the country accepted women. The 1890s and the first half-decade of the twentieth century would see a high-water mark reached for female medical education, with nearly 1,500 women studying medicine each year in the mid-1890s. This point should not be overstated, however, given that from 1890 to 1928 women made up only between 3 and 6 percent of all students enrolled at regular medical schools.[57]

By about 1905, with growing pressure for medical schools to conform to rising standards for curriculum, many medical schools closed or merged, including most of those for women. By 1909, 14 of the nation's 17 women's medical schools had already been shuttered, and the number of women studying medicine decreased to only 921 that year.[58]

One of the more significant debates over women in medicine surrounded the issue of midwifery. Their work in child delivery was largely uncontroversial until the 1880s, when a pair of factors converged to make this a heated debate. Since colonial times, and earlier, midwives had provided a routine presence at child births, particularly for poor and rural women. Among African Americans, birth attendance by a physician was rare, with an estimated 90 percent of all black births attended by a midwife, not by a doctor, even through the 1930s.[59] Physicians had begun attending a greater percentage of births in the early 1800s, particularly in urban areas, but midwifery continued as a standard practice among recent immigrant and rural women and the poor. As late as the end of the nineteenth century, most American births were attended by midwives.[60] Given the diminishing visibility of midwives among the economically stable, white population through the 1800s, their scrutiny was minimal.[61] Attention increased, however, when the second major wave of European immigration in the late 1800s expanded the population of recent arrivals, people who were accustomed to, shared a language with, and were able to afford midwives.[62]

Male physicians, who by this time saw themselves as comprising a professionalized group that enjoyed significant social status, pushed back strenuously against this new infusion of midwives. During the very late 1800s and early 1900s a common view among male physicians was that midwifery was a "necessary evil," necessary because there simply were not enough doctors to attend to every birth.[63] As an interim step, many doctors came to believe that midwives should be better trained and licensed before being allowed to practice. Typical of the period were comments by a physician, writing in 1916, that midwives are, "except in rare instances, ignorant, untrained, incompetent women, and some of the results of their obstetric incompetence are unnecessary deaths and blindness of the infants, and avoidable invalidism, suffering and death of the mother." The solution, in this author's view, was more training, and that "since the evil for this moment cannot be eradicated, the danger to the public can be minimized by some provision for the proper regulation, supervision, and control of the midwife by the state and for her training to do her work in a cleanly and intelligent manner."[64]

As the nineteenth century closed, physicians expanded their presence to attend to approximately one-half of all deliveries, though their presence did not immediately depress rates of maternal death. Child delivery continued to be a dangerous activity. Even as late as 1917 the U.S. Children's Bureau reported that child birth killed more women of child-bearing age each year than any other cause, save tuberculosis.[65] In the short-term, physician-assisted deliveries introduced a new set of problems, such as misused forceps.[66] Due to the ratio of pregnant women to physicians, midwifery continued its significant presence in American medicine, though most states began to regulate or at least monitor their activities. Massachusetts alone outlawed midwifery, in 1907, a move that does not appear to have reduced midwives' activities. New York City required their licensing beginning in 1914.[67] By 1930 only 10 states required neither licensing of midwives nor their registration. These early-twentieth-century legal steps did not silence the debate over midwifery, a debate that has carried on to the present day.[68]

RACE AND AMERICAN MEDICINE

African American physicians struggled for recognition and places to apply their skills throughout the nineteenth century in contexts dominated by white, male doctors. Having emerged from the ranks of herbal healers in the early 1800s, a few black doctors received formal medical training in Europe and began American practices as early as the 1830s.[69] James McClune Smith was among the first, receiving an MD from the University of Glasgow in 1837. The first African American graduate of an American medical school received his MD from Rush Medical College in Chicago in 1847. By 1860 at least nine American medical schools, all in the North, admitted black students.[70] Beyond difficulties gaining admission to medical schools, African American physicians were routinely denied privileges to practice in hospitals, both in the North and in the South. Of course, black patients were often denied hospital admissions well into the twentieth century. Poverty, combined with reduced access to medical services, translated to markedly poorer health outcomes for African Americans from the time such figures began to be kept in the nineteenth century.

A major step forward for black students seeking medical education came with the establishment of Howard University's medical school, open to both black and white students, in 1869. At its beginning Howard began classes with only five faculty and eight students, and it had to contend with resentment from the faculty at Georgetown University across town owing to the competition for white students, and a few faculty, that Howard created. Medical school options expanded gradually through the remainder of the 1800s, and by 1900, 14 other black medical schools had opened, of which most were proprietary schools. Others were church-sponsored. This flourishing of educational opportunities for African Americans was short-lived, as nearly all of these schools either failed or merged with others by 1925 due to pressures put on medical schools throughout the country during the first couple of decades of the twentieth century regarding orthodoxy of curriculum.[71]

Another venue from which African American physicians were generally excluded was the AMA. This issue climaxed in 1869, when doctors Charles Purvis and Alexander Augusta, both military doctors during the Civil War and later faculty members at Howard University, were denied membership in the AMA. Despite protests from at least one member of Congress, Senator Charles Sumner of Massachusetts, the AMA remained intransigent and issued a public letter in 1870 insisting that admission to the AMA was a matter at the Association's discretion. Senator Sumner responded by introducing a bill to revoke the AMA's charter. The bill was unsuccessful, and the AMA continued to deny admission to black doctors. At the AMA's 1870 convention a group of physicians belonging to the Washington, D.C.–based National Medical Society, an organization of black doctors, were refused seating by the majority of the AMA's Committee on Ethics. Dr. Nathan Davis, the historic organizer of the association, found himself in the majority voting to exclude the black doctors.[72] The Association's leadership insisted that the black doctors were excluded because the National Medical Society accepted members who were not licensed to practice, a sin of which the AMA itself was guilty at the time.[73] This episode prompted the creation of the National Medical Association, a nationwide professional association for African American physicians.[74] The AMA explicitly refused to direct its constituent organizations to cease using race as a disqualifier for membership as late as the 1940s.[75] Some local medical societies continued to exclude black members into the 1960s. The AMA issued a formal apology to African Americans in 2008.[76]

These discriminatory factors, combined with widespread poverty among the nation's African American population, meant that rates of infectious diseases, still birth, and various illnesses were significantly higher among blacks than among whites throughout the late 1800s and well beyond. Typical of figures from the early twentieth century, shown in Table 1.1, were those presented to the American Public Health Association in 1913 by Dr. Lawrence Lee.

Lee, a public health department employee in Savannah, took a highly condescending approach, to put it mildly, toward the health of African Americans in Georgia. He noted that "the health of the whites cannot improve unless the health of the colored also improve" and that the blacks need, therefore, better schools, hospitals, and outpatient clinics. Lee continued, noting that "by themselves the negroes will not better themselves. Where they came from they were savages, left to themselves they remain little better than savages. Their nature is such that benefits such as public charities provide, have to be given to them, almost forced on them." With help, "the negro . . . may be made a better citizen. . . . Instead of being a burden he may come in time to look after himself. Whites have to help blacks improve their health so that blacks don't financially drag down the white community."[77] Of course, cross-race disparities in a wide range of health outcomes have continued to plague minority groups up to the present.

ADVANCES IN MEDICAL SCIENCE AND MEDICAL EDUCATION

The late nineteenth century, the leadership of the AMA hoped, would be a time of consolidation of political and professional power for regular physicians. But this was not to be. Arguments at various levels continued into the 1910s over representation of various medical sects on public boards and

Table 1.1
Rates of Illness and Still Births among White and Black People, Savannah, Georgia, 1913

	Rate per 100,000 population	
	White	*Black*
Still births	48	230
Pneumonia	32	84
Bronchopneumonia	6	16
Tuberculosis	48	135
Influenza	3	20

Source: Dr. Lawrence Lee, presentation to the American Public Health Association, Jacksonville, FL, November/December 1914; quoted in Gamble, ed., *Germs Have No Color Line* (Garland 1988).

medical school curricula. One venue where this conflict played out was the creation of local and state health departments. In the 1860s and 1870s most states created state-level health departments.[78] How the directors of these bodies were selected provided a perspective on the conflict between secular and regular physicians. Kansas's example illustrated this difficulty. Kansas sought to create a health department in the early 1870s, but it was delayed due to arguments between practitioners as to how each group would be represented on the board. The solution came in an agreement that no single group would hold a majority. Instead, the governor appointed three regulars, three eclectics, and three homeopaths each year.[79] This level of inter-sect conflict persisted for several decades more.

The conflict between secular practitioners and mainstream medicine was largely put to rest as a result primarily of two factors in the late 1800s and early 1900s. First, mainstream medical science produced a series of breakthroughs in the understanding of disease causation and cures during this period. The development of effective anesthesia during the 1850s so that patients no longer need to die of shock during surgery, learning the value of antisepsis through the 1860s, and the spread of hospital-based laboratories and X-ray machines during the 1890s all contributed to important strides in medical science.[80] As Lawrence Henderson would later famously note, it was not until the second decade of the twentieth century that "for the first time in human history, a random patient with a random disease consulting a doctor chosen randomly stood better than a 50–50 chance of benefitting from the encounter."[81] In light of the resulting progress, it became increasingly difficult to argue persuasively on behalf of practices and education that turned on fundamentally different premises from those of mainstream medicine. Advancements in medical education also occurred during this period. While inconsistency and sometimes low-quality educations persisted throughout the first quarter of the twentieth century, formal medical education began to mark the discipline. This episode, centered on an evaluation of all of the medical schools in the United States, by a taskforce headed by Abraham Flexner, marked a turning point in American medical education.

The editors of the *Journal of the American Medical Association* wrote in 1901, "It is to be hoped that with higher standards universally applied their number will soon be adequately reduced, and that only the fittest [medical schools] will survive."[82] The rapid growth in the number of medical schools troubled the AMA leadership, not only because of the concerns about quality but also because of the financial impact these new schools were having on the field. During the first decade of the twentieth century, many editorials in the *Journal of the American Medical Association* noted that there were "too many schools . . . turning out too many graduates to make practice profitable."[83]

Complaints about doctors' low salaries had often characterized the medical discourse throughout the nineteenth century. After a half century of very modest accomplishments, the AMA refocused its attention on the state of medical education and on politics.[84] An important step was the launching of a comprehensive study of American medical education, the Flexner Report in 1910, which produced a set of findings that hastened the wave of medical school closures, mergers, and significant curricular reforms.

Abraham Flexner, a schoolmaster from Louisville, Kentucky, headed a committee that visited all of the 155 medical schools—regular and secular—in the United States and 8 in Canada. The Flexner Report graded schools, and those grades directly impacted the schools' ability to recruit faculty and students. This widely read document proved tremendously influential in its call for regularizing medical education and the closure of substandard schools.[85] By 1920, 76 medical schools either closed or merged.[86] While this consolidation trend was already under way prior to 1910, the Flexner Report accelerated it.[87] The report took particular aim at proprietary schools, writing that "such exploitation of medical education is strangely inconsistent with the social aspects of medical practice" and that the modern practice of medicine should strive to better the social good rather than to be a "business to be exploited."[88] The pressure this report created to raise admission standards marked a turning point in medical education. The report resulted in the AMA creating a new set of curricular standards, which were widely adopted by schools and state boards, making the AMA's position effectively binding.[89]

Although the Flexner Report has been celebrated as a great turning point in the quality of American medical education—as one observer put it, a "genteel bombshell"—it also involved some disproportionate pain in certain quarters.[90] The closure of medical schools impacted those educating African Americans heavily, as the disappearance of many poorer and semirural schools limited access to black students.[91] By 1923, the medical schools at Howard University and Meharry Medical College were the only remaining historically black medical schools in the nation.[92] For a group already systematically marginalized in terms of school admission, ability to practice in hospitals, and membership in medical societies, these developments surely were seen as yet another setback. On the other hand, curricular reforms were certainly needed. In the last decade of the nineteenth century, only 63 percent of medical students entered school with an undergraduate degree (compared to 36% at the beginning of that century), and only 44 percent had completed a residency.[93] Medical education still did not uniformly involve formal classes complemented by clinical and lab work, but after the full impact of the Flexner Report and the resulting reforms, this triumvirate became the standard.

By 1930 virtually all medical schools required a college degree for admission, three or four years of graded curriculum, and clinical instruction.[94]

ORGANIZED MEDICINE AS AN EMERGING POLITICAL FORCE: THE AMA

The first half century of the AMA saw few significant political achievements. The consolidation of most practitioners under a banner of regular medicine was due as much or more to advances in medical science than it was to political efforts to marginalize sectarian healers. Further, the AMA leadership chose not to involve the Association in issues beyond those immediately relevant to the profession for the sake of not fragmenting its member support. Some viewed this as a series of lost opportunities, as various social problems affecting public health unfolded throughout the late 1800s unconfronted by the nation's largest association of physicians. The Temperance movement came and went, and the AMA took no position. Crowded, unhealthy tenements arose in cities, and the AMA made only feeble efforts to speak to these conditions. Similarly, it did almost nothing in the face of terrible child labor conditions, nor did it speak on behalf of a congressional bill in 1888 that, had it been successful, would have created a national department of public health to investigate food safety.[95] It was not the AMA that called for reforms in dirty manufacturing trades in the early years of the twentieth century, but rather the American Association for Labor Legislation. It was the American Association for Labor Legislation (AALL) that successfully fought for federal regulations to protect workers in match factories who were widely afflicted with "phossy jaw," an illness caused by exposure to phosphorous.[96] The standard explanation for the AMA's reluctance to become involved in these public and worker health issues is that confronting them required no specialized skills, meaning the work could be left to others.[97]

In its defense, the AMA became a key player, albeit belatedly, during the development of the Pure Food and Drugs Act of 1906 through articles and editorials in the *Journal of the American Medical Association*.[98] Other agitators, including the muckraker Upton Sinclair and his 1906 book, *The Jungle*, also played important roles. For its part, the AMA had adopted a sustained interest in combating unproven nostrums during the late 1800s, even though the *Journal* continued to sell advertising for such products into the first few years of the new century.[99] The 1906 act, despite some loopholes, outlawed the manufacture, sale, or interstate transportation of tainted, adulterated, or falsely labeled drugs, drinks, or food.[100] Seeking to build on this victory and having changed its ways, the AMA pushed hard, though unsuccessfully, beginning in 1906 for the creation of a cabinet level national health department.

By retooling its organizational structure between 1900 and 1920, the AMA solidified its status as the nation's preeminent medical organization. The creation of a Speaker's Bureau in 1911 allowed the Association to meet its growing public relations needs more effectively. The *Journal* gradually became a highly regarded publication to advance the Association's political goals in addition to being a significant scientific venue. Association membership grew from 8,400 in 1900, to 70,000 in 1910, to over 83,000 by 1920. A national charter sought from Congress in the first decade of the twentieth century and ultimately approved by the U.S. Supreme Court in 1916 allowed the Association to operate nationwide as a unified body. Up to that point, the AMA was built on representatives from state medical societies, a fragmented federalist model that undermined its power by limiting its ability to operate outside of its home state of Illinois.[101] That nationwide reach would be exercised strenuously during the late 1910s in opposition to national health insurance.

Once the matter of secular medicine had largely waned during the early years of the twentieth century, a chief political concern of the AMA became the protection of what the Association's leadership saw as emerging interference from governments, particularly actions that might offend the near-sacred ideas of the doctor-patient relationship and free-market medicine. Physicians had long seen themselves not only as socially important healers but also as financial entrepreneurs. A broadly shared ethos of laissez faire that militated against federal or state regulation of professions pervaded the field from its early years. As the medical educator John Shaw Billings noted in a speech to the medical faculty at Yale University in June 1891, "the popular feeling is that in a free country every one should have the right to follow any occupation he likes, and employ for any purpose any one whom he selects, and that each party must take the consequences."[102] The AMA leadership did not, on the whole, reject state licensing of physicians in the early twentieth century, but certainly it successfully advanced the idea that the legitimate practice of medicine should not be the subject of government meddling. As publicly funded programs for particular occupational groups—such as disabled seamen beginning in 1798, former slaves under the Freedmen's Bureau, or military veterans after the two world wars—or for purposes of fighting epidemics, the leadership of the AMA abided these efforts, though it strenuously objected to broader government involvement in healthcare financing.

Organized medicine's objections to government involvement extended to service provision as well. At the turn of the twentieth century, city-sponsored medical facilities, traditionally referred to as dispensaries, moved beyond simply handing out drugs. As they offered more medical treatments, the vocabulary changed and they increasingly became known as clinics.[103] In New York, free clinics provided care for up to one-quarter of the city's population by the 1890s.[104] As one defender of the newly expanded practice noted, "It was foolish to examine children without seeing that they received treatment."[105] However, doctors not affiliated with these free clinics routinely criticized them for giving care at no charge to patients who could in fact afford private physicians. The financial resentment was clear, and local doctors accused the city of practicing "a policy of Socialism" and further characterized the practices as "ruinous to the business of the medical practitioners of the city."[106] Beginning in the 1890s, the AMA and local medical groups waged a successful battle on these dispensaries-become-clinics, leading to their virtual elimination in New York by the time of World War I.[107]

Organized medicine's objection to government financing would play a large role during the early twentieth century, as Progressive Era proponents of national health insurance pushed hard for healthcare coverage as a basic right of citizenship. By the beginning of the 1910s various progressive groups called for federal action to expand health coverage. Interestingly, organized labor was not among them. Briefly, prior to the 1940s labor unions generally wanted to preserve health care for workers as a prize they could claim they won for their membership (more on this in Chapter 2). The financing issue would assume major importance with rising health care, due largely to advancing medical technology. Private health insurance, something that had been attempted unsuccessfully in the 1800s, would not assume a prominent place in the medical landscape until the 1930s. When it did, insurance plans relieved some of the pressure to address healthcare costs, but until then calls for national health insurance would be loud and sustained, if unsuccessful. The broader social insurance movement—a movement that saw the creation of workers' compensation, child labor laws, unemployment compensation, and ultimately the Social Security Act in 1935—swept with it many important policy innovations that protected large swaths of the American public. But health care remained outside the ambit of this movement in a way that illustrated both the ambivalent attitudes of the public and policy makers and the difficulty of launching major social programs while using significantly underdeveloped administrative apparatuses to do so. Health care's failure to catch fire along with other social insurance programs is the story of Chapter 2.

NOTES

1. British Broadcasting Company, "Silent Weapon: Smallpox and Biological Warfare" (available online at http:/www.bbc.co.uk/history/worldwars/coldwar/pox _weapon_print.html; accessed July 10, 2008).

2. Duffy 1990, chapters 1 and 2.

3. Ibid., p. 28.

4. Ibid., p. 25.

5. Rosenberg 1962, chapter 1.

6. Ibid., pp. 82–85.

7. Cassedy 1991, pp. 62–63.

8. Numbers 1978, p. 5.

9. Burrow 1963, p. 3.

10. Budrys 2005, p. 87.

11. Burrow 1963, pp. 3–5.

12. Cassedy 1991, chapter 1; Fishbein 1947, p. 19.

13. These schools included Kings College (1764), which would become the medical school at Columbia University; The University of Pennsylvania (1765); Harvard University (1783); The College of Philadelphia (1765); and The Medical School of Dartmouth College (1798). Fishbein 1947, p. 19.

14. Duffy 1990, pp. 20–22.

15. Klepp 2004; Beck 2004, p. 2139; Cassedy 1991; Ferling 1989.

16. Shryock 1967, p. 5.

17. Ibid., p. 4.

18. Klepp 2004, pp. 63–65.

19. Cassedy 1991, p. 51.

20. Klepp 2004, p. 73.

21. Duffy 1990, pp. 26–28.

22. Klepp 2004, p. 71.

23. Duffy 1990, pp. 54–56.

24. Pierce veto on May 3, 1854, *A Compilation of the Messages and Papers of the Presidents*, vol. 6, pp. 2780–2789 (published by Bureau of National Literature, Inc., New York, 1897).

25. Roemer 1945, p. 147; for excellent treatments of the poorhouse movement, see Rothman 1971 and Katz 1996.

26. Roemer 1945, p. 148.

27. Engel 2006, p. 8.

28. Shaw 2007, chapter 2; Roemer 1945, p. 148.

29. Duffy 1990, p. 92.

30. Ibid., p. 122.

31. Roemer 1945, p. 150.

32. Duffy 1990, p. 59.

33. Roemer 1945, p. 149.

34. Duffy 1990, pp. 167–168.

35. Shryock 1967, p. 17.

36. Hudson 1992, pp. 5–6.

37. Cassedy 1991, pp. 36–37.

38. Ibid., p. 26; Roemer 1945, p. 154; Shryock 1967, pp. 48–49.

39. Shryock 1967, pp. 28–29.

40. Harris 1966, p. 1.
41. Burrow 1963, p. 5.
42. Ibid., p. 5.
43. Beck 2004.
44. Fishbein 1947, pp. 21–22.
45. Ibid., pp. 45–46.
46. Shryock 1967, p. 50.
47. Morantz-Sanchez 1985, p. 49.
48. Walsh 1977, p. 53.
49. Ibid., p. 109.
50. Morantz-Sanchez 1985, p. 52.
51. Ibid., p. 54.
52. Ibid., p. 57.
53. Ibid., pp. 54–55.
54. Fishbein 1947, pp. 82–83.
55. "African American Physicians and Organized Medicine, 1846–1968," a time-line by the AMA (available online at www.ama-assn.org/ama1/pub/upload/mm/369/afamtimeline.pdf; accessed July 15, 2008).
56. Both quotes from Walsh 1977, p. 134.
57. Morantz-Sanchez 1985, pp. 65, 249.
58. Walsh 1977, p. 51.
59. Litoff 1986, p. 4.
60. Cassedy 1991, p. 311; Shryock 1967, p. 50.
61. Shryock 1967, p. 50.
62. Litoff 1986, chapter 1.
63. J. Clifton Edgar, reprinted in Litoff 1986, p. 129.
64. Both quotes from Edgar, reprinted in Litoff 1986, p. 130.
65. Litoff 1986, p. 5; Fishbein 1947, p. 20.
66. Litoff 1986, p. 5.
67. Edgar, reprinted in Litoff 1986, p. 140.
68. See Arney 1982, Litoff 1986, DeVries et al. 2001.
69. Cassedy 1991, p. 30.
70. Morais 1967, pp. 30–31.
71. Ibid., pp. 40–42; Savitt 1992, pp. 67–72.
72. Morais 1967, pp. 53–54.
73. Fishbein 1947, pp. 80–81.
74. Burrow 1963, p. 6; Shryock 1967, p. 51.
75. "African American Physicians and Organized Medicine, 1846–1968," a time-line by the AMA (available online at www.ama-assn.org/ama1/pub/upload/mm/369/afamtimeline.pdf; accessed July 15, 2008).
76. AMA press release, July 10, 2008 (available online at http:/www.ama-assn.org/ama/pub/category/print/18773.html; accessed July 15, 2008).
77. Lee quoted in Gamble 1988, p. 73.
78. Lee 2007, p. 24; Anderson 1985, p. 44.

79. Lee 2007, p. 24.
80. Cassedy 1991, p. 76; Howell 1995, chapter 4.
81. Quoted in Somers and Somers 1961, pp. 136–137.
82. Beck 2004, p. 2139, quoting the *JAMA* editorial.
83. Shryock 1967, p. 57.
84. Burrow 1963, pp. 56–57.
85. Cassedy 1991, pp. 89–90.
86. Hiaat and Stockton 2003; Burrow 1963, p. 36.
87. Hudson 1992, p. 8.
88. Beck 2004, p. 2139.
89. Ibid.
90. Hudson 1992 (quote at p. 7).
91. Beck 2004, p. 2140.
92. "African American Physicians and Organized Medicine, 1846–1968," a timeline by the AMA (available online at www.ama-assn.org/ama1/pub/upload/mm/369/afamtimeline.pdf; accessed July 15, 2008).
93. Hudson 1992, p. 3.
94. Shryock 1967, p. 63.
95. Bremner 1956, especially chapter 5; Burrow 1963, pp. 21–24.
96. Numbers 1978, p. 16.
97. Anderson 1985, p. 45.
98. Burrow 1963, p. 71.
99. Shryock 1967, pp. 71–72.
100. Lee 2007, p. 35.
101. Burrow 1963, pp. 32–33, 45–49.
102. Billings 1891, p. 1.
103. Starr 1982, p. 366; Numbers 1978, p. 5.
104. Duffy 1990, p. 158.
105. Numbers 1978, p. 8.
106. Ibid., p. 8.
107. Duffy 1990, pp. 158–159 (quote at p. 159).

2

Not Quite Catching the Wave: Health Care and the Early-Twentieth-Century Social Insurance Movement

The period from 1910 to the late 1930s saw the flowering of America's welfare state in a variety of respects. States adopted workers' compensation and mothers' pension programs, Congress legislated a federal framework for state unemployment programs, and with the passage of the Social Security Act of 1935, Congress created old-age pensions, a federal cash welfare program for the children of single parents, and under later amendments to that landmark act, disability insurance payments for those unable to work. Government-coordinated health insurance, despite strenuous and prolonged efforts by progressive-minded advocates, was not included in this wave of social programming. Some social welfare historians have asserted that the early part of this period, particularly between 1915 and 1917, marked a moment when national health insurance stood a realistic chance of enactment. Although it is true that for a short time the leadership of the nation's most politically active medical society, the AMA, did not actively oppose the idea, that posture did not endure, and throughout this period several other forces took a clearly negative view toward government-mandated health insurance. Organized labor divided on the question, with the influential American Federation of Labor opposed well into the 1920s. Southern members of Congress disapproved of how national health insurance might unsettle race relations, and even erstwhile allies of the reformers were skeptical of the administrative apparatus proposed to implement such a program. Complicating matters, Woodrow Wilson took little interest in health insurance during his administration, World War I blocked any grand plans for domestic policy making, and by the time Franklin Roosevelt became president, organized opposition was so fierce that national health insurance appeared to stand so little chance of enactment that he declined to invest much of his political capital in it. Harry Truman was the first president to endorse compulsory insurance unambiguously, but by the late 1940s various forces blocked any such effort, including a well-funded public relations campaign against it, the rise of private insurance that undermined the apparent pressing need for it, and a time of Republican control of Congress that severely limited the liberal agenda. Thus, despite several significant expansions of America's welfare state, social insurance has remained incomplete, lacking a way to address the healthcare needs of working-age people who cannot afford private insurance. This chapter examines this period with particular attention paid to the key moments of the 1910s, the mid- to late 1930s, and the late 1940s, times when campaigns for national health insurance were most active.

PROGRESSIVE ERA EFFORTS TO ENACT NATIONAL HEALTH INSURANCE

American progressives drew no small amount of inspiration from European adoptions of sickness insurance for workers. Germany led the way with its enactment of government-organized insurance in 1883, followed by Austria in 1888, Hungary in 1891, Norway in 1909, Serbia in 1910, Britain in 1911, Russia in 1912, and the Netherlands in 1913.[1] These plans for compulsory health insurance involved mandatory participation by workers and their employers, with financial contributions by each, subsidized by national governments. Given that 33 U.S. states had adopted worker's compensation programs by 1916, beginning with New York in 1910, adopting compulsory health insurance appeared as a logical next step in worker protection.[2] Both found their justifications in notions of enlightened capitalism. The sooner a worker is made healthy, the more productive he or she will be.

The economic context of the 1910s favored conversations about extended worker protections. Growing economic displacement of the American working class, with urban populations expanding from 19 to 45 percent of the nation's population between 1860 and 1910 and the nonagricultural labor force dropping from 69 to 42 percent, fostered a sense that theories of individual responsibility could no longer explain why so many workers fell ill or suffered disabling injuries that kept them out of the labor force. Progressives on the leading edge of campaigns for broader social insurance justified this move as a way of enhancing individual freedoms, but what they were actually doing was calling for limits on the freedom of industrialists to pursue their own individualistic goals in order to improve the material security of their employees.[3]

This call for a government-sponsored safety net marked a fundamental change in thinking. Capturing the essence of the movement, one social insurance advocate declared that "our conception of the function of the State is changing. . . . The well-being or ill-being of the individual is now looked upon as a social asset or liability and not simply as a matter of personal concern alone to the individual."[4]

Regarding medical care in particular, early-twenty-first-century Americans tend to think of its provision as having a primary goal of helping the population maintain sound health, a good in itself. However, early efforts to advance workers' compensation and sick pay turned at least as much on economic stabilization as on maintenance of good health per se. Among the European nations that adopted compulsory health insurance, it was not the more liberal polities but rather the more authoritarian ones that were the early innovators. Germany's case saw the monarchy in the 1880s, sensing threats from its political enemies, and Bismarck envisioned government health care as a way to secure workers' loyalty.[5] Theodore Roosevelt, though not necessarily to be compared too closely to Bismarck, advanced similar thinking in his Progressive Party Platform of 1912, which proposed "the protection of home life against hazards of sickness, irregular employment and old age through the adoption of a system of social insurance adapted to American use."[6] This was the first time that compulsory health insurance was endorsed by a major party.

Striving toward economic stabilization was important, but it was complemented by a sense that recent great medical strides should be shared widely and that improvements in medical technology could readily facilitate this. Viewing poor health as a primary cause of poverty, successful human interventions against diseases and illnesses became particularly appealing.[7] By 1910, medicine had made remarkable progress. The plagues of the previous century were either eliminated or were well on the way to being controlled.[8] Improving public health came to be seen as a way to strengthen the nation as a whole. As the British Prime Minister Lloyd George put it, "You cannot maintain an A-1 empire with a C-3 population."[9]

Efforts at private insurance were attempted in the second half of the 1800s but were unsuccessful. Several private insurers in the 1850s suffered bankruptcy, and later attempts in the 1890s involved policies issued to cover specific illnesses, but these were costly and appealed mainly to the middle class.[10] With private health insurance not particularly viable, medical technology advancing, and a mature awareness of the health impacts on worker productivity, by about 1910 the political logic of a campaign for government-coordinated insurance seemed clear, providing what seemed like an opportune moment for advocates to add it to a growing safety net.

THE PROGRESSIVE ERA AND A MODEL BILL FOR GOVERNMENT-ORGANIZED HEALTH CARE

Central to the history of the Progressive Era struggle for national health insurance was the AALL, a group of social progressives formed in 1906 to lobby for legal reforms. These progressives were not radicals and their ranks included prominent mainstream figures such as Louis Brandeis, Woodrow Wilson, Roscoe Pound, Jane Addams, Samuel Gompers, and Edward Devine.[11] After its victory in the first decade of the twentieth century on behalf of workers in the match factories and the success of workers' compensation plans in the states, the AALL organized the nation's first conference on health insurance in 1913. That gathering and their work the following year produced a model piece of legislation for compulsory health insurance, which it published in 1915.[12] Under the title Health Insurance—The Next Step, the Association's bill provided for surgical, medical, and nursing insurance for injured workers to receive a cash benefit during their absence from work for up to 26 weeks (benefits were to be worth two-thirds of a worker's pay), pregnancy services for insured women and the wives of insured men, and a $50 funeral benefit. The state would pay 20 percent, the employer 40 percent, and the worker 40 percent. The bill borrowed ideas from the German and, to a much lesser extent, British models.[13] The model bill did not call for universal coverage, rather only for workers and their dependents. The need to address the economic impact of lost wages was significant, as illustrated by a 1919 study of several thousand workers in Chicago that found one-fourth of workers sick that year, typically missing more than a week of work, with lost earnings averaging nearly 14 percent of one's annual wages.[14] Reflecting its strategy of working within white, middle-class norms of the day, the model bill did not cover agricultural workers and domestics, which had the effect of excluding about 5 million workers in the latter group, half of whom were African Americans.[15]

At its outset in 1915, the campaign for the state adoption of the AALL's model bill enjoyed moderated support of the AMA, with many in its leadership believing that some sort of compulsory health insurance was probably inevitable, given the wide adoption of health insurance in Europe and because many members of the AMA appeared supportive of the cause. Prior to 1910 the *JAMA* had run editorials critical of European compulsory insurance plans, but recognizing its likely adoption in the United States the *JAMA* noted that American doctors should present a "united front and a moderate but positive" attitude in order "to secure a living income before the inadequate compensation offered has become crystallized into legislation."[16] Once the push was under way in the United States, the AMA's Committee on Social Insurance reported that "blind opposition, indignant repudiation, bitter denunciation of these [compulsory insurance] laws is less than useless; it leads nowhere and it leaves the profession in a position of helplessness as the rising tide of social developments sweeps over it."[17] Further, a pair of 1916 editorials in *JAMA* took the position that "no other social movement in modern economic development is so pregnant with benefit to the public" and that "much of the best informed opinion of the country is in favor of these proposals . . . which ought to result in an improvement in the health of the industrial population and improve the conditions for medical service among the wage earners."[18] Others in the medical profession, including Michael Davis, director of the Boston Dispensary, supported the idea and believed that the concerns he had over the potential for inappropriate bureaucratic control of doctors could be obviated by local insurance committees negotiating with individual doctors or small groups of them.[19]

It would be an overstatement to attribute the AMA's endorsement of the model bill to an enthusiastic approval by rank-and-file members, many of whom may have indeed been agnostic toward the proposal. A late 1916 survey of secretaries of state medical societies revealed that the large majority of them had not yet discussed health insurance with their membership, and despite chapters in Wisconsin and Pennsylvania having endorsed it, others encountered strong opposition.[20] Much of the resistance was economic in nature. A 1911 editorial in *JAMA* took a dim view of contract medical purchasing, as was then occurring among some fraternal organizations and mutual aid societies. Critics lambasted this practice as "buying a physician's services at wholesale and selling them at retail" and that this amounted to medical exploitation.[21] In a context where the AMA leadership believed that only a small minority of doctors earned a comfortable income, it was understandable that the Association would adopt a cautious approach to the details of payments under any compulsory insurance bill.[22] In short order, certainly by the middle of 1916, the matter of wages and the feared implications of the model bill became a stumbling block for many doctors. The question of how physicians would receive payment—either at a capitation rate involving a set payment per worker subscribing to the plan or by a fee-for-service arrangement—would need to be settled. European experiences had revealed that fee-for-service arrangements likely would lead to public budget problems, but American doctors were reluctant to commit to a capitation system, given that this might drive competition between medical providers.[23]

Before the opposition reached full strength, the AALL's bill was introduced in 15 state legislatures. It received particular attention in New York and California. In the latter, the state's social insurance commission recommended the adoption of compulsory insurance in the early 1917. This prompted a group of doctors to form an opposition group, The League for the Conservation of Public Health, that took the view that compulsory health insurance was "a dangerous devise, invented in Germany, announced by the German Emperor from the throne the same year he started plotting and preparing to conquer the world."[24] Ad hominem charges evoking the specter of an oppressive or socialist state would become common surrounding health care by the beginning of World War I, but they were evident before then as well. California voters defeated compulsory health insurance in a 1918 referendum.[25]

Many critics of the New York version of the bill, the Mills bill introduced in early 1916, focused their objections on what they perceived to be short-comings of the legislative language much less than on the idea of compulsory insurance per se. The problem, according to these critics, was that too little attention was given to ensure that physicians could earn a reasonable living under the proposed system. The Medical Society in Manhattan called for the provision of a minimum wage for doctors participating in group contracts and the stipulation of the number of people to be enrolled under these agreements. William Gottheil, a noted dermatologist, wrote of the Mills bill in New York that it "would rob a hard-working and well-deserving body of citizens [i.e., physicians] of a large part of their means of livelihood."[26] In 1918 the California League for the Conservation of Public Health argued publicly that the plan would "emasculate the medical, dental and pharmaceutical professions, and pauperize or bankrupt the members."[27] In hindsight, many in the medical profession regretted not opposing the bill more straightforwardly from the beginning. To have not mounted a vigorous opposition to the bill from its outset led some AMA leaders to look back years later on their indecision during 1917 as their "single greatest mistake."[28]

Another important dimension of the New York debate over the model bill turned on its presumed impacts on organized labor. Samuel Gompers, president of the American Federation of Labor during the 1910s, strongly opposed government involvement in health care out of his belief that labor unions did better to negotiate the good of their workers instead of relying on a paternalistic state to do so. Gompers called the AALL's insurance proposal "a menace to ... [the] rights, welfare, and liberty" of American workers.[29] He worried that "a government insurance system would weaken unions by usurping their role in providing social benefits."[30] This was the overshadowing problem. Due to an underdeveloped sense of class consciousness in the United States, labor unions faced enough challenges without ceding potential prizes to the state. As Gompers saw it, "the unions desired to develop their own system of protection against all the vicissitudes of life as a means of gaining recruits. Social security would deprive them of that function."[31] Others had also come to see the state as no friend of organized labor, such as Warren Stone of the Locomotive Brotherhood, who commented that he did "not believe in a government that tucks you in bed at night."[32]

As significant as the American Federation of Labor was, Gompers's view did not characterize those of all in the larger movement or even those of the AFL leadership by the mid-1920s.[33] The New York State Federation of Labor, the American Association of Wire Weavers Protective Association, the Women's Trade Union League, and the International Ladies' Garment Workers' Union all supported the model bill in New York. The latter two joined on once maternity benefits were added to the bill, but their initial hesitation clearly arose from a different place than Gompers's objections. Female laborers at the time tended to take a more collective welfare approach than did their male counterparts.[34]

Across the nation, insurance companies comprised another source of resistance to compulsory health insurance. They saw it as a direct threat to their business, particularly the bill's inclusion of a death benefit for workers, a slice of the market that insurance companies viewed as lucrative. In 1917 several life insurance companies came together to form the Insurance Economics Society of America in order to pool their opposition to the AALL's proposed legislation.[35]

Between crystallizing opposition by state medical societies, the AMA, and the insurance companies and the lack of a unified voice from organized labor, the AALL's bill faced long odds by 1917. If these obstacles were not enough, the onset of World War I sealed the movement's fate. Ideas originating in Germany became increasingly suspect, as reflected in the comment by one Maine physician that "whatever comes to us labeled 'Approved in Germany,' should be carefully examined beneath its wrappings to see if there be not concealed a Prussian."[36] When the California League for the Conservation of Public Health asked rhetorically in 1918, "What are we fighting for 'over there'? We are fighting for our American birthright—principles of equality and personal freedom—inalienable rights, that we must not forfeit here for this mess of German pottage—Compulsory Health Insurance."[37] Widespread popular misunderstandings of how compulsory health insurance might work fostered suspicion of imported policies. By the end of the war, support for government-organized healthcare financing had so eroded that the AMA's 1920 formal statement opposing it was much less of a controversial move than it would have been three or four years earlier. Within this short time the idea of compulsory health insurance had been so dragged through the mud and associated with German-ness and Bolshevism that it was hard to imagine, in many quarters, it being resurrected as a viable political campaign. In 1925 the New York Medical Society noted that "it is not conceivable that any serious effort will again be made to subsidize medicine as the hand-maiden of the public."[38] They were right, for the moment.

It is important to note that during this time the overwhelming share of the political efforts to legislate compulsory health insurance unfolded in the states, not at the federal level. Although some aspects of federal policies certainly exhibited an activist government throughout the late 1800s and early 1900s—Civil War pensions were one, regular annual appropriations to fund Indian health care beginning in the 1910s were another—there still existed a strong and widespread sense that the Constitution simply did not provide for federal social insurance policy-making authority. Advocacy of bold plans for national health insurance would have to wait until conditions changed in the 1930s.

THE CHANGING FOCUS OF REFORMERS' EFFORTS IN THE 1920s

One important development during the 1920s was the growing awareness of the need for health insurance as a response to rising medical costs, not simply as a way to fill the gap left by lost wages. To the reduced extent progressive reformers continued to work on their compulsory insurance plans during the 1920s, they encountered a changing environment regarding healthcare economics. Previously, lost wages had typically exceeded the cost of the associated medical services, but with technological advances this situation had changed. Medical care had become more expensive, doctors raised their fees to recoup their own higher educational costs (brought on by more rigorous curricular standards), and expectations for medical services had increased. The result was that nonwealthy people faced a new obstacle to health: the high cost of seeing a doctor.[39]

Physicians in the 1920s tended to respond to rising costs by giving ground in two important respects. First, they came to welcome government construction of hospitals and clinics, an activity that would see significant expansion throughout the 1940s and 1950s, even amidst continued robust opposition to government involvement in healthcare financing. Second, realizing the growing gap between medical costs and poor patients' ability to pay, they came to moderate their opposition to government reimbursements for care of the medically indigent. The second point did not develop easily, as many doctors resented the Sheppard-Towner Act of 1921, which offered federal grants to states to cover basic health and hygiene services and education for mothers and their infants, and a 1924 veterans program. Federal reimbursements were not precisely the problem, but rather that the fees paid were set not by doctors but instead by the government. Many physicians believed this was an invasion of the doctor-patient relationship and that the program would steer patients toward doctors participating in that program and away from purely private practice physicians.[40] The AMA continued its opposition to Sheppard-Towner during the mid-1920s. The program was ended in 1927, and later attempts to resurrect it met with more heated rhetoric from the AMA, calling such efforts in 1930 "unsound . . . , wasteful and extravagant, unproductive of results and tending to promote communism."[41] Resentments notwithstanding, the AMA tolerated the veterans' program, as it provided a way for former service members to become patients, where in the absence of federal funds, many of them would not have been. In the case of the veterans' program, the numbers were substantial, nearly 1.4 million from World War I.[42]

By the late 1920s the two major camps—liberal reformers versus the AMA—had adopted completely incompatible positions. Various causes drove this breakdown in discourse, but the greatest was the clash of beliefs between those who thought that well-functioning citizens required some measure of economic and health security and those conservative opponents who instead saw supreme justice in the market. Another part of this growing divide turned on doctors' self-image. As Daniel Hirshfield's history of this era notes, "Most doctors of this period probably saw themselves as engaged in the most difficult profession in the world. They were daily called upon by society to take human life in their hands and pit their skill against illness and death. In return, society accorded them high social status. Individual doctors took satisfaction in their work and its social prestige: this was the ideal reward of the medical profession; incidental financial success was not."[43]

FAILURE TO LAUNCH: NO NATIONAL HEALTHCARE LEGISLATION IN 1935

During the 1920s and the early years of the Great Depression, the rising awareness of how many Americans could be considered medically indigent softened opposition to federally sponsored welfare medicine. This was not to pronounce the death of notions of economic individualism, for even in 1935 the Gallup poll found that 60 percent of respondents believed too much was being spent on relief.[44] However, to an extent, individuals' inability to purchase the medicine they needed rendered the medical assistance programs for the poor more palatable. In the early 1930s New York State had established, under its Temporary Emergency Relief Administration, a program to pay for medical services for the poor. Franklin Roosevelt carried the broad outlines of this program with him into the presidency and incorporated them into the work of the Federal Emergency Relief Administration. There were certainly points of resistance, but this federal experience, which ended in 1935, taught doctors and advocates lessons, principally that government involvement in medicine could proceed without disaster. This opened the door to further public-sector roles, but these experiences also reinforced the awareness on the part of doctors that they, not government bureaucrats, should maintain dominant control.[45]

The main push for government-organized health insurance occurred in the second half of 1934 and into 1935. Roosevelt's Committee on Economic Security (CES), formed in June 1934, was charged with developing the legislative language that would, the following year, become the Social Security Act. Various cabinet secretaries along with prominent academics made up the CES, including Secretary of Labor Francis Perkins, Director of the Federal Emergency Relief Administration Harry Hopkins, economist Edwin Witte, social policy expert Arthur Altmeyer, the prominent health insurance reformer Edgar Sydenstricker, and his staff assistant Isidore Falk, among others.[46]

Some of the senior members of the CES, including Hopkins, favored a government-organized, mandatory approach to health insurance.[47] Despite his closeness to the president, Hopkins's idea would be left untried. Throughout this period Roosevelt's endorsement of compulsory health insurance was tepid. From the beginning, the president and his secretary of labor had essentially concluded that the CES should not consider health as part of the initial package of proposals. Altmeyer later wrote that "the committee recognized that this was a very complex and controversial subject which might jeopardize speedy and favorable congressional action on its other recommendations" of the Social Security bill.[48] Roosevelt's fear of derailing old-age pensions led him not only to temper his public rhetorical support for national health insurance but also to instruct the CES to omit any health provisions from the bill he sent to Congress. Sydenstricker, it seems belatedly, realized in the spring of 1935 that health provisions would not be included in the developing bill, so instead he convinced the CES to include a statement that healthcare needs continued to be pressing and were being considered by the committee.[49] Word of the study caught the attention of the AMA, which in turn generated a large number of protests to the White House and Congress from doctors opposing compulsory insurance. Witte remarked, referring to the single sentence in the bill calling for the study of health care, "that little line was responsible for so many telegrams to members of Congress that the entire social security program seemed endangered until the Ways and Means Committee unanimously struck it out of the bill."[50] Sydenstricker and Falk had viewed the language of a study as a possible strategy to bring doctors into the conversation, hopefully with the goal that their protests would subside. The AMA's leadership, however, was in no mood to be co-opted.[51]

The mood of the leadership of the AMA, in fact, was one of fierce opposition to further steps toward compulsory insurance. Morris Fishbein, the editor of *JAMA*, noted in an editorial in March 1934 that the threats of socialized medicine posed by such programs surely involve "hundreds of thousands of bureaucratic employees who idle through their six-hour days; they see them snooping into the intimacies of American family life, coming between the doctor and his patient, and waxing fat on the tax money extorted from wage earners and employers alike."[52] With this attitude on public display, it is hard to imagine why certain administration figures envisioned cooperation with the AMA.

Once the CES's report surfaced with its principles for thinking about next steps toward national health insurance, the AMA responded by developing its own set of 10 principles within which its leadership believed the political conversation should unfold, including freedom of choice, aid directed only at the poor, and other limitations on program scope. Apparently Sydenstricker mistakenly thought that the presence of these principles implied that the AMA was still serious about sitting down with reform advocates to find common ground. The AMA had no such interest in mind.[53] Instead, the *JAMA* ran a series of editorials in February 1935 opposing government health insurance. The AMA's House of Delegates, in June 1935, approved a two-year program by the Association's Committee on Legislative Activities "that was designed to defeat any 'trial horse legislation' which the reformers might introduce."[54] The AMA's oppositional efforts were effective, in part because they played against an internally divided Committee on Economic Insecurity.

In 1934 and 1935 other medical groups were not so opposed as was the AMA. The American College of Surgeons had endorsed national health insurance at its recent conference, held shortly before a late 1934 national conference convened to consult on the Social Security bill.[55] Despite their voices, however, by the spring of 1935 Roosevelt asked his CES to drop any formal call for health insurance from its final report and instead to merely mention it as a possible future direction. All accounts indicate that Roosevelt was afraid that due to the AMA's opposition, the presence of a health plan in the report would shoot down the larger Social Security plan. He did not want to run that risk.[56] Congressional Democrats seemed to take a similarly cautious approach, as the Ways and Means Committee reported when it passed the rest of the Social Security Act in April. It included some federal funds to advance public health but noted that public health services "should not be confused with health insurance," a step it was not willing to take at the time.[57]

Edwin Witte, in his postmortem on the Social Security Act, wrote that "it was my original belief . . . that it would probably be impossible to do anything about health insurance in a legislative way, due to the expected strong opposition of the medical profession."[58] Writing in 1963, Witte had the benefit of considerable hindsight, specifically of political battles ranging over more than three decades, experiences that would have reinforced his impression of the impossibility of comprehensive health legislation. For the moment, he was right, even if two years later, in 1965, he would be disproved. Government approaches to health through Witte's time in government had taught him that progress tends to come in piecemeal fashion, with various New Deal programs involving small healthcare components. Emblematic of the incremental style of contemporary American politics, these fragmentary efforts reflect twentieth-century healthcare provision then and now.

UNSUCCESSFUL ATTEMPTS TO AMEND THE SOCIAL SECURITY ACT: 1937-1939

The political actors committed to national health insurance in the mid-1930s saw openings between 1937 and 1939 to add a comprehensive health benefit to the Social Security Act. Their optimism would turn out to be misplaced, and their enthusiastic campaign would help cement the opposition from the mainstream medical establishment and from those whose concerns stemmed from fiscal conservatism or virulent anticommunism. The broad arguments for and against compulsory insurance through the late 1930s differed little from those used during the 1934–1935 effort, with the exception of shifting debates about the extent of federal versus state involvement. In the main, language of health care as a basic right of citizenship dueled with that of a slippery slope toward socialized medicine. Unhappily for liberal reformers, President Roosevelt offered little rhetorical support, and solidifying fears about a slide into socialism created a potent obstacle to shifting the debate to terms that might resonate more powerfully with the American public.

The starting point for this round of the conversation was the research and bill drafting undertaken by the president's Interdepartmental Committee on Health. A subgroup, the Technical Committee, addressed specific features of a proposal for compulsory insurance. Unfortunately for its members, the Technical Committee's National Health Program was watered down to a collection of very general ideas when the time came for the larger committee's report to be produced in February 1938. This downgrading of a plan for compulsory insurance from its greater status in 1934 undermined any chance of specific pieces of the plan to get much political traction. The Technical Committee's idea of tying federal health grants to states to a requirement that states adopt a compulsory insurance scheme won little support among senior administration staffers, and once those two ideas were uncoupled, compulsory health insurance became an even lesser priority for the administration than it already was.[59] As one notable account put it, "Compulsory health insurance was thus seriously enfeebled by the time the Technical Committee finished its final report in February 1938. It had been segregated and insulated from the other recommendations of the National Health Program, assigned the lowest priority, and couched in the least specific terms. . . . The administration was apparently once again willing to sacrifice this reform on the grounds of political expediency."[60]

This weak administrative support—a long-standing theme and part of the institutional explanation for why the United States has no national health insurance—was, of course, only part of the problem for reformers. Contrary ideas also played a key role in thwarting efforts in the late 1930s to enact a comprehensive health policy. Opponents continued to attack government-organized health insurance on both a broad level and in some very particular ways. In the former sense, they argued about the feared impacts on patients' freedom of choice, and on the doctor-patient relationship more generally, and the notion that public-sector medicine would turn doctors into disempowered agents of the state. In narrower senses, they voiced concerns that too much federal involvement would interfere with the autonomy of states and that it would subordinate doctors to nonmedically trained government bureaucrats.

For their part, medical societies did not consistently line up with the AMA. Dissension within the medical community complicated the building of broad coalitions. In 1937 a group of 430 physicians had parted ways with the AMA to call for a national health policy that would address all segments of the nation's population.[61] By this time there also existed a Committee of Physicians for the Improvement of Medicine, numbering some 400. These "medical New Dealers" produced a 1937 document of "Principles and Proposals" proposing a tax-funded national health policy. In the spring of 1938 the president of the American College of Physicians spoke out against what he called the AMA's "partisan behavior" in its opposition to a national health policy.[62] Nonmedical groups, such as the NAACP, and various farming and urban constituency organizations testified before Congress during this period, taking the position of health care as a basic citizenship right.[63]

In the summer of 1938 proponents of national health insurance gathered at the National Health Conference in Washington, D.C., organized by the Interdepartmental Committee staff, and with Roosevelt's blessing, some 150 delegates representing farm and labor groups, business associations, government agencies, health professionals, and others met to discuss ideas for what they saw as a way forward.[64] The meeting produced a set of recommendations, including the expansion of existing federal public health services, enlargement of federal grants for hospital and clinic construction, greater federal assistance to state medical care systems for the medically needy, a worker disability benefit program to temporarily replace a portion of wages lost to injuries, and a general program of medical care, paid for either through general taxation or through social insurance contributions.[65] Excluding the disability and health insurance components, the Technical Committee estimated the cost to be $850 million annually, once fully phased in over a decade. Most of the plan's proponents believed that this approach would bring about greater financial efficiency in healthcare delivery.[66]

In a move that was perhaps calculated to avoid seeming obstructionist but also reflecting the AMA's gradually growing acceptance of public health care for the poor and of public grants for physical infrastructure, the AMA House of Delegates offered support for four of the National Health Conference's five points, excluding the call for a plan for general health insurance. Apparently sensing more political controversy than he wanted to tackle at the moment, the president asked the committee to shelve the National Health Program for the time being. A few months later, in January 1939, Roosevelt sent the Conference's proposal to Congress with a brief note attached urging enactment. He did little else to push matters along.[67] The president told Arthur Altmeyer, who chaired a group within Roosevelt's CES, early that year that he did not intend to make health care a major piece of the congressional campaign in 1938 but that he would return to it in his own reelection campaign of 1940.[68] In a context of the beginning of the war in Europe, the political flack Roosevelt took for his failed court-packing plan, and the growing disenchantment by rural and Southern members of Congress over his urban and welfare-focused efforts, the president's decision to delay what would need to be a major policy proposal was understandable, especially given his uncertainty about fighting the medical lobby over this issue.[69]

Without Roosevelt fully on board, Senator Robert Wagner of New York introduced a bill calling for national insurance in February 1939.[70] This was the first of what would be several versions of a compulsory health insurance bill sponsored by Wagner and his Senate colleague James Murray of Montana and House Member John Dingell, Sr., of Michigan.[71] The bill called for the establishment of medical assistance to mothers and infants, an expansion of federal funds for the U.S. Public Health Service, increased federal funding for hospital and clinic construction, and the launch of a temporary disability payment program. All the bill's provisions could be adopted by states voluntarily.[72] Some reform allies, such as the Committee of Physicians for the Improvement of Medical Care, supported the bill, but the opposition both within and without the medical community was adamant and well organized.[73]

Hearings began on the bill in Senate committee in April 1939. A host of erstwhile supporters of the bill exhibited both an overall affinity and misgivings about the proposed administrative structures. Their testimony inadvertently raised doubts. Medical groups opposing Wagner's bill challenged it head-on, expressing irritation that the bill could be interpreted to allow the construction of government-owned hospitals that would compete with their own, among other objections. The AMA launched a negative publicity campaign, citing high government costs and vagueness of language, criticizing the overly strong federal role, and raising fears that it would destroy state and local initiatives. After several months of hearings and consideration and still facing this opposition, in June 1939, Senator Murray tabled the bill. By December, Roosevelt had shifted his support away from the Wagner-Murray-Dingell bill to an alternative that supported hospital construction, a move that must have seemed more comfortable than going to the mat for a comprehensive bill he thought would prove unlikely to secure.[74] The hospital construction proposal was ultimately passed after squabbles over the question of how much ongoing federal aid would be available to communities that were arguably too poor to maintain them. Those looking for the aid got most of what they wanted. This program, dubbed the "Fifty Little Hospitals Bill" by those who thought it too modest, must have seemed like a blessing to the AMA and the American Hospital Association, since it represented federal financial backing without any further interference in the practice of medicine.[75] A hospital and clinic construction program was a far cry from what proponents of comprehensive legislation wanted. It is impossible to say whether a more vigorous effort by the Roosevelt administration would have achieved this more ambitious end.

THE RISE OF VOLUNTARY HOSPITAL AND PREPAYMENT PLANS

If government involvement in healthcare financing posed what seemed to some in organized medicine a dire threat, this public-sector invasiveness was not the profession's only problem in the 1930s and 1940s. The market-driven development of voluntary hospital and prepayment plans, what would become Blue Cross and Blue Shield, posed an interesting challenge to staunch opponents of anything other than individually negotiated fee-for-service arrangements or private commercial insurance. The first of these voluntary, collective efforts to finance and deliver medical services dates to the 1890s, when railroad, lumber, mining, and other companies operating far from settled communities, along with mutual aid societies, contracted with individual physicians or small groups of doctors to provide care for all their workers or members on a per-capita charge basis. Building on this collective model, the first nonprofit, secular hospital opened its doors in Dallas in 1929. By the early 1930s group hospitalization arrangements operated in communities across the nation. These prepayment plans varied. Some were limited to particular groups, such as occupational groups; others were open to members of

entire communities or users of a particular hospital. Elaborating and formal-
izing these approaches were the Blue Cross (hospital services) and Blue Shield
(physician care) plans dating from 1937.[76]

Voluntary plans challenged opponents of group contract financing because
they invited medical providers into systems that offered set fees for each patient
in the group, limiting what doctors could charge, and yet these collective programs enticed providers to join by promising access to large pools of patients
whose office visits were backed with guaranteed payment from the plan. Because
these plans were not creatures of government, the tempting charge of socialized
medicine did not quite stick (though some used it anyway).

Responding to this changing environment, the AMA highlighted the financial constraints such plans posed for doctors. As early as 1926 the AMA's Judi-
cial Council warned, "It goes without saying that for any organization of any
kind to offer for an agreed stipend more than the reasonable worth of that
which is offered is wrong in principle, and physicians should guard themselves
against being connected with such organizations."[77] Clearly, the AMA saw the
rise of voluntary associations as a dangerous development. When the editor of
JAMA reflected on these growing organizations in the March 1933 edition, he
wrote that the failure of these associations to include the services of all doctors
and hospitals in a certain area opened the door for compulsory health insurance.[78] Walter Reuther, the vice president of the United Auto Workers, told
the story of a doctor who was willing to sign a contract with Blue Cross in his
area. "The medical society launched a propaganda campaign that charged that
it was socialism. We pointed out that the government was not involved at
all. . . . Two weeks later, one of our doctors asked for his contract back. He said,
'My wife and I are both being ostracized socially, and they're threatening to take
away my hospital privileges.' "[79] Physicians in other parts of the country who
cooperated with prepayment plans faced "blacklists, denials of hospital privileges, and accusations of unethical practice."[80]

Although these voluntary plans were seen as problematic by many in the
medical profession because of their violation of the traditional private negotiation of fees between medical providers and patients, their proponents held up
Blue Cross plans as designed in part to defuse further calls for government-
organized medicine. Walter Dannreuther, an early Blue Cross organizer,
declared that Blue Cross would "eliminate the demand for compulsory health
insurance and stop the reintroduction of vicious sociological bills into the state
legislature year after year."[81] The rapid expansion of these plans and private
insurance more generally gave the middle class less reason to agitate for a
public-sector solution to the gaps in health coverage for Americans.[82]

Critics notwithstanding, the move to voluntary associations marked a
shifting of terrain that simply would not be stopped. By 1937, 21 Blue Cross

plans operated in at least 11 states.[83] During the 1930s the AMA surveyed businesses and leaders of state medical societies to poll their opinions on such associations. The responses were overwhelmingly positive.[84] Not all state medical societies took such favorable views, however. The District of Columbia Medical Society and the AMA itself were charged in 1938 with violating federal law in their attempts to inhibit the nonprofit Group Health Association, Inc. In what the U.S. Justice Department believed was a violation of the Sherman Anti-Trust Act's restraint-of-trade provision, the District of Columbia Medical Society had threatened to expel any doctor who served on the board or participated in medical consultation with the Group Health Association. The ruling in the federal district court favored the medical societies, but on appeal the ruling went against them, as did the decision by the U.S. Supreme Court in 1943. The resulting $2,500 fine paid by the AMA constituted a minimal financial setback, but it represented a loss of prestige for the Association.[85] In response, by the mid-1940s the AMA leadership began to limit its complaints about voluntary associations trying to insist that they were most appropriate to service poor people who might otherwise have no access to medical providers. Recognizing how widespread the voluntary associations were and that there was no legal way to stop them, the AMA ceased its active opposition to voluntary associations.[86] By 1946 Blue Cross plans covered some 20 million people in 43 states.[87]

State governments were also brought into the equation, and they recognized these voluntary, nonprofit plans with favorable legislation and court opinions, starting with New York's legislation in 1935. This law served as a model for many other states that adopted similar statutes throughout the remainder of the 1930s. Given their unique status as nonprofits, the question arose as to whether they should be regulated similarly to for-profit insurers. Nearly half the states answered that question in the negative and passed laws governing them but also exempting them from taxation and the conventional requirements of substantial cash reserves that apply to other insurers. Other states insisted on taxing these plans, as they did commercial insurance companies. By the early 1940s nearly all the states had adopted legislation governing the Blue Cross and Blue Shield plans.[88]

For their part, not all medical providers complained about prepayment plans. The American Hospital Association was a significant catalyst behind the rise of Blue Cross. Further, many doctors appreciated the enhanced ability of a broader clientele to meet their expenses. These plans seemed to work especially well in rural areas where patients were traditionally serviced in charity fashion due to their lack of insurance. By the early 1940s, some 20 million Americans were covered by some 210 different prepayment plans.[89]

The spread of insurance plans, whether profit-driven or not, added another layer of complication to the debate over healthcare financing during the middle part of the twentieth century. As private insurance companies developed a larger stake in market outcomes, they took more aggressive efforts to pressure policy makers. This was still a time when most expenditures on health in the United States were private, either out-of-pocket or donations from foundations to hospitals and research. Later, the balance would shift toward more public than private money flowing into health, and that would change the debate in still other ways.

With Roosevelt no longer willing to fight for compulsory health insurance, a significant growth of private and nonprofit insurance programs under way, and a growing agreement that federal aid to hospital construction was a politically winning strategy, the 1940s opened with a sense on the part of many reformers that this new decade would be one of incremental attempts to expand medical coverage. With a divided administration and an organized opposition, grand strides toward a national healthcare plan seemed unlikely to succeed.[90] This did not dissuade liberal Democrats from pursing various versions of Senator Wagner's bill, but their efforts would prove unsuccessful.

The conversation about the need to address public health was recharged in the early 1940s when approximately 40 percent of the first million men drafted for World War II were found to be either mentally or physically unfit for military service.[91] While this generated a certain amount of public and congressional interest, it did not change the fundamental terms of the debate.[92] Neither did the 1942 release of the Beveridge Report, a British plan for cradle-to-grave social insurance that its namesake, Sir William Beveridge, touted during a U.S. tour as a model not only for his own country but also for Americans. Some liberal sources, such as journalist Richard Stout in *The New Republic* in December 1942, characterized national health insurance as a valuable step toward the creation of an American social minimum. Stout believed the "Beveridge Report is the firecracker that will finally startle the public into contemplating the matter."[93]

Some of the public tuned in to the debate, with polls through the mid- to late 1940s typically finding between one-half and two-thirds of respondents reporting having heard or read about the proposed legislation.[94] Organized medicine did much more than merely tune in. The years 1943 and 1944 saw the AMA organize to fight government health insurance, opening an office in Washington, D.C., in 1944 and running a steady stream of articles in its *JAMA* in order to alert allies of the continuing threat of federal legislation. Dr. Morris Fishbein, *JAMA*'s editor, undertook a multicity speaking tour in addition to his editorial work against the Wagner-Murray-Dingell bill, arguing that if Congress passed federal legislation the powers of the

U.S. Surgeon General might exceed those of Hitler.[95] Fishbein's history of heated rhetoric dated back to the 1920s, when he had used the editorial page of the *JAMA* to paint those who agitated for compulsory insurance as being guilty of "incitement of revolution."[96] Fishbein's emotionalism eventually led to his removal as the *JAMA*'s editor, but the Association's leadership did not temper its intransigence against what it saw as the danger of socialized medicine. The AMA's campaign during the mid-1940s employed a pamphlet, among others, titled "$3,048,000,000 of Political Medicine Yearly in the United States" that characterized the Wagner-Murray-Dingell bill as a step that, if taken, would demote doctors to mere public employees who would work only eight hours a day, and that emergency patients would need to wait until the work day started before being seen. Exaggerated as it was, the fear-mongering likely contributed to continued opposition to the bill.[97]

The two sides had settled into their respective positions, with lobbyists for organized medicine arguing that further government involvement in financing would lead to lay bureaucrats encroaching on territory that rightly belonged to physicians and with pro-government activists arguing that a national policy would not only enhance the efficiency of healthcare expenditures but also improve public health through more comprehensive coverage. Doctors tended to argue for their professional autonomy as trained providers, whereas opponents often accused medical societies of merely circling the wagons for the sake of defending turf. *The New Republic* opined in 1943 that "As long as organized medicine in the United States continues to shirk its public duty while fighting a defensive battle against what it regards as lay encroachment upon its province, so long will both doctors and their potential patients suffer, and so long will the nation pay a gigantic bill for preventable disease."[98] Roosevelt's presidency came to an end without him ever being able to close the deal with Congress on what many New Dealers saw as the missing piece of America's social insurance coverage.

HARRY TRUMAN'S PUSH FOR COMPULSORY HEALTH INSURANCE

Upon assuming the presidency, Harry Truman announced compulsory health insurance to be a priority.[99] Wasting no time, in the spring of 1945 Truman signaled his support for the latest version of the Wagner-Murray-Dingell bill. Owing to a lack of support among senators from rural states and the South, the bill achieved little traction. The administration's continuing urban focus had alienated some Democrats whose votes might have helped the bill along. Undaunted, Truman delivered a radio address to the nation in November 1945 devoted entirely to health care. Beyond calling attention to various problems with public health and related issues, the president proposed federal grants to help build hospitals and clinics and expanded services targeted at women and children.[100] For the first time, national health insurance advocates believed that they had a strong ally in the Oval Office.[101]

Pursuing what was probably the least controversial component of his plan, in 1946 Truman called for the passage of the Hill-Burton Act, a hospital construction grant program that would become his only significant legislative accomplishment in health care. The need to improve the country's stock of hospitals was compelling. The number of hospitals had risen throughout the 1920s, reaching some 4,300 in 1928, but had then declined during the Great Depression, falling back to only about 4,000 in 1935. As of the late 1940s in the United States, there was only one general hospital bed for every 263 persons. Cross-state disparities were dramatic. In 1948 New York had one bed for every 196 persons, compared to one per 667 persons in Mississippi. Some 1,300 of the nation's counties had no hospitals at all.[102] Under the act, states received grants and distributed them to cities, towns, and counties. This much was not particularly controversial. However, problems arose in connection to the conditions attached to the grants. As a nod to segregationists, racial discrimination was permitted where equal facilities were available nearby. The U.S. Supreme Court struck down the separate but equal provision for hospitals in 1963.

In an effort to extend care for the poor, facilities that received Hill-Burton funds were expected to provide what was referred to as a reasonable volume of free care each year to the poor. (Compliance provisions were not written into federal law until 1979.) Because grants were distributed on a dollar-for-dollar matching basis, wealthier communities were able to take advantage of the program more readily than poorer ones, and because local sponsors—either municipalities or not-for-profit organizations—had to demonstrate that they possessed the resources to maintain the facilities, relatively few of the nation's poorest communities took advantage of the program.[103] Southerners insisted on and won deference to state practices, meaning that the legislation allowed states to decide who would be served at the new hospitals and who would be allowed to practice medicine there, which allowed states to continue excluding black doctors and patients or segregating them as they had historically done. During the debate, Alabama's Lister Hill proposed that on the question of "Who shall practice in the hospitals, and the other matters pertaining to the conduct of hospitals, we have sought in the bill to leave to the authority and determination of the states, and not have the federal government, through this bill, invade the realm of the operation and maintenance of the hospitals."[104] The legislation required hospitals to sign a nondiscrimination contract, but the law also explicitly allowed for racial segregation as hospitals saw fit. Early on, North Carolina availed itself of the segregationist option under its Hill-Burton grant and constructed a pair of all-white hospitals, a pair of hospitals for blacks, and 54 other facilities that were racially segregated by ward.[105]

On the more challenging bill, that sponsored by Wagner, Murray, and Dingell, hearings did not produce the outcomes progressives had hoped for. Early in the proceedings, Ohio Senator Robert Taft began an argument with Senator Murray about whether the bill was socialistic. He went on to tar Murray's earlier full-employment bill as having "come straight out of the Soviet Constitution" and that the current bill was, to Taft's mind, "the most socialistic measure that this Congress has ever had before it."[106] Taft became so agitated in the course of this dustup that he stormed out of the hearing, clearly indicating that Democrats could not count on Republican votes for the measure.[107]

Beyond arguments about socialism, fears of bloated government bureaucracies were evoked by such groups as the American Dental Association, which promoted the belief that the Wagner-Murray-Dingell bill would create "the greatest bureaucracy the world had ever known."[108] For its part, the American Hospital Association called for expanded private insurance as a way to extend access. Amidst these competing arguments, by mid-1946 the fight for the bill was essentially over. Murray announced in July that he would not pursue the bill more at the time but rather after that year's November elections. Interparty rivalries, personality conflicts (by this time Taft was probably already thinking of running for president in 1948), emerging red-baiting, and more general resistance from conservatives within and beyond Democratic Party ranks made for an inhospitable political context for any compulsory health insurance legislation.

It was during these first couple of postwar years that President Truman failed to follow up on his earlier forceful positions regarding the need for greater government involvement in health care. Throughout 1946, he spoke publicly about this issue only three times. Archival records indicate that the president had not lost interest—he continued to follow developments—but he became oddly reticent on a topic on which he had been quite outspoken in 1945. Apparently his sense of that he could not match Roosevelt's rhetoric or the welter of conflicting events nearly silenced him regarding health care.[109]

A lost opportunity or not, the political season in 1946 ended with congressional elections that returned Congress to Republican control. Backlash against Truman in particular and the New Deal/Fair Deal more generally lay behind the outcome. Republicans ran under the slogan "Had Enough?" in 1946, and it worked. Republicans came into power in Congress in 1947 with their own bill, this one much more limited than the Democratic version and focused on federal grants to participating states to fund medical services for the poor, grants for cancer research and for periodic screening of children, and the creation of a federal health agency to organize health-related activities.[110] To qualify for government-funded services, individuals were required to satisfy a means test to validate their neediness, a move that was political anathema to liberal Democrats. Sensing the political danger of legislating a partial fix, a move they rightly feared would placate many moderates for years to come, Senator Murray criticized the GOP measure as "relief medicine, through public charity." Congresswoman Helen Gahagan Douglass of California called it an "insult to the dignity of our self-supporting, self-respecting American people."[111] Senator Wagner reiterated his call for "adequate medical services on the basis of need, not ability to pay," which he argued was the "birthright of every American."[112] Republican Senator Taft was not moved and indicated his belief that health care was like any other commodity; only those who are unable to participate in our free-enterprise system should receive it from government at no direct cost. Given the very real possibility of a Truman veto, the Republican bill probably never stood a realistic chance of becoming law, but the shift in the conversation turned out to be significant in the long run. Despite the president's arguments that a much broader swath of the population needed public medical aid, including not only the poor but also the elderly, Republicans stood by their argument only for charity medicine.[113] This more limited coverage approach would find its ultimate expression in the 1965 enactment of Medicaid.

Beyond the substantive debate over competing approaches to improved access to medicine during the late 1940s were the symbolic arguments that, in an era of an emerging Cold War and a potent anticommunism, carried considerable weight. Charges that government involvement in health care constituted socialized medicine, far more often hurled than explained, were not new, but as the 1940s reached a close they came into sharp focus. Several high-profile espionage trials elevated fear of socialist subversion to a fever pitch. This context made linking Truman's health proposal to these perceived dangers highly effective.

A central character in this crusade was Marjorie Shearon, a former employee of the U.S. Public Health Service under Isidore Falk. Her 1947 pamphlet, "Blueprint for the Nationalization of Medicine," and an article in the *American Journal of Public Health* attempted to tie all those who supported a national healthcare policy to a communist plot headed by Falk himself. Shearon labeled these people "collaborationists, fellow-travelers, appeasers, satellites, and gullible accepters."[114] Shearon, as an aide to Senator Robert Taft, provided direction for Senate Republicans in questioning those testifying on health legislation before moving on to work for the Republican National Committee in a similar capacity. In her rendering of the communist network, what she called the "House of Falk," the central conspiracy behind national insurance flowed from the leftist International Labor Organization. Shearon propagated these charges in numerous addresses to conservative groups during the late 1940s, portraying Falk as an evil genius who controlled people in various executive branch agencies and did the bidding of the International Labor Organization in the United States. She further insisted that the Wagner-Murray-Dingell bill was not really a domestic product but rather a document written by staff at the Geneva-based labor organization.[115] Falk, in his later appearance before congressional committees, systematically dissected Shearon's inaccuracies about him and his work, dismantling the alleged International Labor Organization links. However, his efforts to show that Shearon did not have her facts straight did little to neutralize the charge of socialized medicine.[116]

Before ending his presidency, Harry Truman considered an alternative approach to consensus building, one that reached out to the AMA and other opponents. Truman revisited his earlier tactic of highlighting the deficiencies of public health. With work by Oscar Ewing, the administrator of the Federal Security Administration, a study was undertaken of the nation's health needs. Ewing arranged for a meeting of representatives from health providers, organized labor, farm organizations, and consumer groups at a National Health Assembly. It came together in February 1948, and the outcome was a pleasant surprise to the AMA, whose leaders presumed that the gathering would be stacked against them. The assembly's final report stopped short of calling for national insurance. Instead it proposed that voluntary health insurance, not a compulsory or a single-payer system, could broaden coverage far beyond the bounds envisioned in Senator Taft's bill and in a way that avoided a means test. As it turns out, the proposal satisfied too few Republicans due to its ambition and fell short for many congressional Democrats still intent on more. Truman's declining popularity and his criticisms of the eightieth Congress as the do-nothing Congress did little to advance the proposal.[117]

The 1948 elections returned Congress to Democratic control, but Truman's rocky relations with members limited his influence among a rank and file that had generally grown weary of his agenda. Still sensing danger, however, the AMA board of trustees vowed to exhaust the group's treasury if need be in order to defeat Truman's comprehensive health insurance program. Needing more funds, it levied a $25 per member fee that would fund the Association's campaign.[118] The $1.5 million of AMA money paid to the public relations firm Whitaker and Baxter sufficed in a context already unfavorable to Truman's idea to maintain the sense that increased government involvement in medicine was an inappropriate strategy.[119]

Part of Truman's problem was Truman himself. When asked in public opinion surveys between 1945 and 1950, solid and sometimes quite large majorities of Americans professed support for both the broad ideas that Truman believed in and the Wagner-Murray-Dingell bill. In 1947 and 1948, polls found that more than 80 percent of respondents "believed the government should make it easier for all people to have access to medical care," and only 29 percent believed that it would be a "bad idea" to support national health insurance.[120] But when asked about particular provisions, such as compulsory employer contributions, support waned. In 1949 a Gallup poll found the public divided on this question, with 44 percent supporting salary deductions and 47 percent opposing them.[121] When asked in 1949 if they favored or opposed Truman's plan, respondents who had heard of it divided evenly, with 38 percent favoring and the same percentage opposing it (25% had no opinion).[122] When asked the same question in November 1950, only 30 percent supported Truman's plan, while 57 percent opposed it.[123] Regarding the bill sponsored by Wagner and his colleagues, the primary resistance seemed to reside in Congress and among the various highly active interest groups opposed to the bill, not with the general public. A Gallup poll in April 1946 had found that 55 percent of those who had heard of the Wagner-Murray-Dingell bill favored it. Fewer than 30 percent opposed it.[124]

Looking back, Arthur Altmeyer's digest of the period suggests that in 1946 the Truman administration might have found common ground with Senator Taft through a charity medical grants approach. Altmeyer, having been a lead Truman administration official in social policy, explained that the reason for not seeking that solution was that to do so would have limited the federal assistance to aid to the medically needy, leaving uncovered middle-class people who might suffer unexpected medical crises.[125] Altmeyer was right about the implication of legislating welfare medicine. The year before his 1966 book was published Congress had done just that in the form of the Medicaid program, though it had also created Medicare for retired workers of all income levels. These developments, discussed in Chapter 4, set the United States on a path—characterized by layers of charity medicine for the poor and little else in the way of government assistance for nonpoor Americans of working age—from which it has not departed. Perhaps desperate for some sort of progress in expanding coverage at the middle of the twentieth century and frustrated that the wave of social insurance expansion that marked the Progressive Era and the New Deal had not included comprehensive health legislation, Democrats shifted tactics and pursued government care for the poor. A decade later, such efforts would gain a serious foothold on the policy landscape in the form of the Kerr-Mills program. Whether viewed as caving in to staunch market-oriented opposition or simply adopting a dose of political pragmatism, progressive-minded reformers found a new path near the end of the Truman administration, one that would indeed improve access to medicine but which would leave uncovered a great portion of Americans.

NOTES

1. See Starr 1982 for a comprehensive introduction to early medicine and the United States as a social insurance laggard, especially Book 2, chapter 1.

2. Rubinow 1916, pp. 1–2.

3. Hirshfield 1970, chapter 1.

4. Numbers 1978, p. 14.

5. Starr 1982, pp. 238–246.

6. Numbers 1978, p. 15.

7. Oberlander 2003, p. 18.

8. Numbers 1978, p. 1.

9. Starr 1982, p. 239.

10. Ibid., pp. 241–242.

11. Hirshfield 1970, p. 12.

12. Starr 1982, p. 244.

13. Numbers 1978, pp. 25–26; Stevens and Stevens 1974, p. 9.

14. Starr 1982, p. 245.

15. Funigiello 2005, p. 16.

16. Numbers 1978, p. 30.

17. Oberlander 2003, p. 19.

18. *JAMA* quotes from Oberlander 2003, p. 19, and Burrow 1963, p. 144, respectively.

19. Starr 1982, pp. 247–248.

20. Ibid., pp. 248–253.

21. Burrow 1963, p. 140.

22. Numbers 1978, p. 9.

23. Starr 1982, p. 248.

24. Ibid., p. 253.

25. Fein 1986, p. 37.

26. Numbers 1978, p. 65.

27. Ibid., p. 80.

28. Hirshfield 1970, p. 19.

29. Hoffman 2001, p. 115; see also Starr 1982, p. 249; Cassedy 1991, p. 71.

30. Starr 1982, p. 249.

31. Ibid., pp. 249–250.

32. Hoffman 2001, p. 129.

33. Poen 1979, pp. 19–20; Hoffman 2001, p. 118.

34. Hoffman 2001, pp. 115–120.

35. Hirshfield 1970, pp. 21–22; Starr 1982, pp. 251–252.

36. Numbers 1978, p. 77.

37. Ibid., p. 80.

38. Ibid., p. 109.
39. Starr 1982, pp. 258–260.
40. Hirshfield 1970, pp. 33–34.
41. Burrow 1963, p. 162.
42. Starr 1982, pp. 258–260; Burrow 1963, pp. 152–153.
43. Hirshfield 1970, p. 39.
44. "Do you think expenditures by the government for relief and recovery are too little, too great, or just about right?" (Gallup, September 10–15, 1935; based on approximately 1,500 personal interviews)
45. Hirshfield 1970, pp. 81–82.
46. Ibid., p. 45; Altmeyer 1966, p. 7.
47. Poen 1979, p. 17.
48. Altmeyer 1966, p. 27.
49. Hirshfield 1970, p. 52.
50. Oberlander 2003, p. 21; quoting Feingold 1966, p. 91.
51. Hirshfield 1970, p. 46.
52. Quoted in Burrow 1963, p. 203.
53. Hirshfield 1970, p. 62.
54. Ibid., p. 66.
55. Witte 1963, p. 180.
56. Poen 1979, p. 17; Hirshfield 1970, pp. 44–49.
57. Funigiello 2005, p. 20.
58. Witte 1963, p. 174.
59. Hirshfield 1970, pp. 102–108.
60. Ibid., pp. 107–108.
61. Funigiello 2005, p. 29.
62. Ibid., p. 31.
63. Ibid., p. 43.
64. Hirshfield 1970, p. 108.
65. Proceedings of the National Health Conference, 1937, pp. 29–32; Poen 1979, p. 19.
66. Hirshfield 1970, p. 111.
67. Poen 1979, pp. 22–23; Hirshfield 1970, pp. 115–117.
68. Altmeyer 1966, p. 96.
69. Poen 1979, p. 23.
70. Bill # S. 1620.
71. Oberlander 2003, p. 21.
72. Hirshfield 1970, pp. 139–140.
73. Funigiello 2005, p. 41.
74. Hirshfield 1970, pp. 143–146, 154.
75. Ibid., pp. 157–158; see also Funigiello 2005, p. 46; Poen 1979, p. 24.
76. Richardson 1945, chapter 2; Rorty 1939, p. 211; Law 1974, chapter 2; Fein 1982, chapter 2.
77. Richardson 1945, p. 80.

78. Burrow 1963, p. 230.

79. Quadagno 2005, pp. 24–25.

80. Starr 1976, p. 69.

81. Rothman 1994, pp. 14–15.

82. Fein 1986, chapter 2.

83. Anderson 1985, p. 123.

84. Richardson 1945, p. 87.

85. Burrow 1963, pp. 247–249. See *The American Medical Association v. United States* (1943).

86. Burrow 1963, pp. 250–251.

87. Roemer 1945, p. 162; Anderson 1985, p. 124.

88. Anderson 1985, p. 126; Richardson 1945, chapter 5; Law 1974, chapter 2; Fein 1986, chapter 2.

89. Law 1974, chapter 2; J.D. Ratcliff, "Health for the Back Woods," *The New Republic*, vol. 106, #23, June 8, 1942, pp. 789–791; "U.S. Medicine in Transition," *Fortune*, vol. 30, #6, December 1944, pp. 156–164, 186, 188, 190, 193.

90. Poen 1979, p. 25.

91. Ibid., p. 30.

92. Ibid., p. 31.

93. Richard Strout, "The Beveridge Report," *The New Republic*, vol. 107, #24, December 12, 1942, pp. 784–786 (quote at p. 785).

94. In 1949 Gallup asked, "Have you heard or read about the Truman administration's plan for compulsory health insurance?" 66 percent said yes, 34 percent said no. (November 27–December 2, 1949; based on approximately 1,500 personal interviews)

95. Poen 1979, p. 46.

96. Hirshfield 1970, p. 33.

97. "U.S. Medicine in Transition," *Fortune* 1944, pp. 186, 188.

98. "The Health Program," *The New Republic*, vol. 108, #16, April 19, 1943, pp. 531–532 (quote at p. 532).

99. Poen 1979, pp. 53–55.

100. Speech text available online at www.presidency.ucsb.edu/ws/print.php?pid=12288 (accessed May 15, 2008).

101. Poen 1979, pp. 64–65.

102. Budrys 2005, p. 45; Carl Malmberg, "The State of the Nation's Health," *The New Republic*, vol. 118, #18, May 3, 1948, pp. 15–19.

103. Starr 1982, pp. 348–351; Marmor 1999, p. xxiv.

104. Quadagno 2005, p. 78.

105. Ibid., pp. 78–79.

106. Poen 1979, p. 88.

107. Funigiello 2005, p. 68.

108. Poen 1979, p. 89.

109. Ibid., pp. 70–74, 91–92.

110. Ibid., p. 96; Funigiello 2005, pp. 70–71.

111. Funigiello 2005, p. 70; see also Poen 1979, pp. 96–97.

112. Poen 1979, p. 97.

113. Ibid., pp. 100–101.

114. Ibid., p. 109.

115. Derickson 1997.

116. Funigiello 2005, p. 72.

117. Poen 1979, pp. 117–122, 126–127.

118. Ibid., p. 142; Altmeyer 1966, p. 171.

119. Poen 1979, p. 162; Funigiello 2005, p. 81.

120. Figures from Steinmo and Watts 1995, p. 343.

121. "Should the U.S. Congress pass the government's compulsory health insurance program which would require wage or salary deductions from all employed persons to provide medical and hospital care for them and their families?" (Gallup, May 2–7, 1949; based on approximately 1,500 personal interviews)

122. "What is your opinion about it—are you for the administration's plan, or not?" (Gallup, March 6–11, 1949; based on approximately 840 personal interviews with those who had heard of Truman's plan [56% of all respondents])

123. "What is your own opinion about it—are you for the administration's plan, or not?" (Gallup, November 12–17, 1950; based on approximately 716 personal interviews with respondents who had heard of the Truman plan [48% of all respondents])

124. "What do you think of this bill?" (Gallup, April 12–17, 1946, based on personal interviews with approximately 645 respondents who said they had heard of it, 43% of all respondents)

125. Altmeyer 1966, pp. 261–262.

3

Policy Growth without a Plan or Philosophy: The 1950s and Early 1960s

The 1950s represented a time of change in health politics in two important respects. First, private health insurance became widespread, with more than a tenfold increase in the percentage of the workforce covered during this decade. This growth, together with opposition from the Eisenhower administration, blunted calls for broad, government-based insurance. Second, because the growth of employer-based health insurance did not tend to cover retirees, the growing sense throughout this decade that the elderly increasingly needed assistance meant that opposition to government help with health care for this part of the population lost much of its moral force. Arguing against benefits for the elderly poor—people who had struggled through the Great Depression and who had carried the nation through World War II—became increasingly difficult from a political perspective. As most of the elderly did not benefit from employer-based insurance once they retired, changes in the insurance market left them largely exposed to the challenges of aging and the rising cost of medical services. The inauguration in 1950 of federal payments to reimburse medical providers who extended services to the poor helped some but not all opponents to see that government involvement in the medical market was not simply a slippery slope toward socialism.

These developments would, by 1960, position health care as a top-shelf issue in a presidential election year. With this momentum, even before Kennedy's ascendance to the presidency, government health care for the aged took a significant step forward with the passage of the Kerr-Mills program in 1960, which extended and formalized the federal reimbursements enacted a decade earlier. In 1961, with Democrats firmly in control of both elected branches, the conversation gained even more momentum, and almost immediately following the elections of 1964, with an even more liberal Congress on its way to Washington, the last of the resistance to Medicare and Medicaid would be broken.

This chapter traces two developments—government insurance and the increasingly visible plight of the elderly—during this period of transition of the healthcare debate. It was a time of incremental moves, seemingly without much concerted direction or philosophy. Only in hindsight did it become clear how events would condition the creation of Medicaid and Medicare in 1965, the most significant health policy changes in the nation's history. In the end, three levels of medical coverage—outpatient physician services, hospital care, and assistance to the poor—were combined into a single legislative package that created new entitlements for the aged and those of modest means. This achievement marked a proud moment for advocates who had fought for years for government insurance. That victory, however, did not fundamentally change the conversation about medical insurance for working-age, nonpoor people, as resistance to government involvement in the healthcare market certainly persisted. In hindsight, the Republican strategy of means testing and targeting government health assistance prevailed. Instead of government involvement in the healthcare market being a slippery slope over which doctors are demoted to mere public employees, the relatively narrow scope of Medicare and Medicaid has remained largely intact and has, as Democrats feared in the late 1940s, taken much of the wind out of the sails of those who sought universal coverage. Thus, as is often the case, small steps do not appear to exert much impact while they are being taken, but in hindsight, choosing one path rather than another set a mold for American healthcare policy that would powerfully condition the possibilities during the 1960s and still limit options at the beginning of the twenty-first century.

THE RISE OF PRIVATE INSURANCE

One of the more important developments in healthcare financing during the first half of the twentieth century came with decisions in 1943 by the National War Labor Board and the Internal Revenue Service, later codified in law in 1954, that employer contributions to employee benefit packages would not be counted as wages.[1] This twofold benefit allowed employers to deduct the cost of health insurance from their profits, reducing the portion of earnings subject to federal taxation, and it provided workers with a tangible increase in the value of their compensation packages without boosting their tax obligations. From employers' perspectives, the change also allowed them to build worker allegiance and potentially to head off further calls for unionization.[2] Labor unions tended to see greater security through bargaining, including health care, as opposed to security through government benefits.[3] As these factors converged during the late 1940s and into the 1950s, the number of privately insured workers grew from approximately 1 million in 1947 to 12 million in 1957, plus their 20 million dependents.[4] Free market advocates heartily approved of the spread of private insurance, while a substantial portion of the cost was in fact provided by the federal government in terms of foregone revenue.[5]

The tax incentive created in the mid-1940s has generally been viewed as a great stride forward in creating an employer-based health insurance system. However, this change did nothing to help individuals lacking a regular labor force attachment. Persons who sought insurance through charitable organizations or who purchased it out of pocket did not enjoy the same tax break. Hence, the expansion of employer-based health insurance helped those who held steady jobs, but inequalities in the labor market carried over into inequalities in coverage for the self-employed, the marginally employed, and the unemployed.

Private insurance offerings had met with marginal success prior to the 1930s, due in large part to their tendency to cover only catastrophic illnesses, or to be very expensive, or both, limiting their mass appeal. With the rise of Blue Cross and Blue Shield plans, moderate-income people enjoyed another option and flocked to those plans by the millions. By the 1950s, however, private insurers began cherry-picking healthy people from the roles of Blue Cross plans, allowing private, for-profit insurance companies to assert themselves in the market.[6] As opposed to underwriting based on community ratings, treating all members of a broad group or community equally, private insurers adopted experience rating based on the amount of medical services an individual or compact group used in the previous year. Experience rating allowed insurance companies to offer policies carrying lower premiums when they marketed them to relatively healthy clients, luring those people away from Blue Cross and Blue Shield plans, leaving the latter with a less healthy clientele, which in turn forced them to raise what had been quite affordable premiums. By 1958 Blue Cross found itself $40 million in the red.[7] These market changes, though certainly stressful to the nonprofit plans, led to greatly expanded coverage. By the middle of the 1950s, 60 percent of the population had some sort of health insurance.[8]

INSURING THE ELDERLY

The logjam over government involvement in health insurance would eventually be broken by the compelling need to address the medical needs of

America's elderly and the influx of liberal Democrats into elective office in the mid-1960s. Ideas about a Social Security–based plan to cover senior citizens had surfaced as early as the mid-1940s but were abandoned then by Democrats who persisted in believing that by sheer political will they could achieve coverage more universal than might be achieved under the limited reach of Social Security.[9] As the 1950s progressed, the universal strategy gradually gave way to one that instead targeted the elderly as the reality of limited possibilities became apparent. In 1951 a push to enact medical assistance for those on Social Security attempted to leverage sympathy toward the nation's older citizens but was unsuccessful. Truman aide Oscar Ewing noted to a group of reporters in that year that "it is difficult for me to see how anyone with a heart can oppose this [type of program]."[10] The AMA did oppose it, but it also directed most of its attention to combating compulsory insurance in the form of the Wagner-Murray-Dingell bill. In 1951 it spent some half-million dollars on this effort, and another quarter million in 1952. By late 1952 the AMA disbanded its campaign having won the fight, or so it thought.[11]

Repeatedly, conservative and even moderate members of Congress had refused to lend support to bills that would have added a health benefit under Social Security. Such a benefit, if added, still would have left approximately one-half of all those over age 65 uncovered, since they were not Social Security eligible.[12] Part of the explanation for the failure to turn a corner on this debate was found in the halfheartedness of the Democrats. Indicative of this was language in their 1952 party platform that merely affirmed President Truman for attempting to make progress toward "an acceptable solution to this urgent problem."[13] For their part, the Republicans were more specific in their opposition, declaring that they rejected "federal compulsory health insurance with its crushing cost, wasteful inefficiency, bureaucratic dead weight, and debased standards of medical care."[14]

Organized medicine marked the inauguration of Dwight Eisenhower in 1953 with a sigh of relief. The AMA president noted at the time that "as far as the medical profession is concerned there is general agreement that we are in less danger of socialization than for a number of years."[15] When the Congress finally created the Department of Health, Education, and Welfare in the spring of 1953, its first secretary, Oveta Culp Hobby, a Texas Democrat, declared that hers would be "an AMA administration," in contrast to the universal healthcare agenda long advocated by Arthur Altmeyer and Isidore Falk, both of whom found themselves pushed out of government at the beginning of Eisenhower's term.[16] The doctors' lobby had fought Truman every time he had proposed a cabinet-level department to oversee federal health efforts. In contrast, Eisenhower promised to stay out of the AMA's business.[17]

Secretary Hobby quickly developed a reinsurance plan under which 25 million federal dollars would be distributed to private insurance companies to subsidize the risks they would take to issue low-cost health insurance policies.[18] Eisenhower pitched this plan to a gathering of presidents of many of the nation's top private insurers at the White House in 1954 believing that this reinsurance arrangement would help the sale of private policies flourish, once the risks associated with catastrophic coverage could be alleviated. Despite his promise that this was not an attempt to introduce government interference into the healthcare market but rather to partner with private industry, the insurance executives remained unconvinced.

Resistance came from other quarters too. The AMA decried the reinsurance effort as "the opening wedge to . . . socialized medicine."[19] Congressional Democrats opposed it because they thought it represented too much of a giveaway to insurance companies. Senator Murray noted wryly that "President Eisenhower has been getting free, socialized medical care almost all his adult life. It is obvious that there is no reason why he personally would have developed any real understanding of this particular problem."[20] The reinsurance bill was defeated in the Senate by a single vote, partly by Murray's protest, and in the House partly because it offended House Minority Leader Sam Rayburn, a fellow Texan who was irritated at Hobby for accepting a post in a GOP administration.[21] Eisenhower, who was otherwise in near synchronicity with the AMA throughout his administration, on this occasion complained that the AMA leadership was to fault for the legislative failure and that they were "just plain stupid . . . a little group of reactionary men dead set against any change."[22]

Change would indeed come, but years would pass before even a fragile consensus could be built. Of chief importance during the latter half of the 1950s was the growing sense that the health needs of the disabled and the elderly demanded some sort of attention. When the Wagner-Murray-Dingell bill was introduced yet again in 1955, it met with staunch resistance. As the leadership of the AMA geared up to fight it with a public education campaign using even more aggressive rhetoric than that engineered by the public relations firm Whitaker and Baxter, the incendiary tactics initially contemplated led the Association's friends in Congress to counsel moderation, given the gradually evolving public mood on the issue. An AMA official later conceded that had the Association employed this take-no-prisoners approach that "we would have looked awful. Can you imagine going to the public and seeming to argue that it's subversive to give Social Security to a disabled workman? We'd have been tarred and feathered as being against cripples."[23] The ground was indeed shifting. A disability benefit under Social Security was successfully legislated the next year. While the movement was small, the precedent set was significant as it built on the creation of federal grants in 1950 to reimburse medical costs for the poor.[24] More political losses for the AMA would follow.

The achievement of disability pensions under Social Security was partly attributable to the reluctant acknowledgment by liberals that an incremental strategy may indeed prove successful. The leadership of the AMA noted the dangers of confronting an incremental strategy, and Elmer Hess, a former president of the organization, wrote Eisenhower in 1956 after the president signed the Social Security expansion complaining that "Truman was easier to handle because he came at you head-on. . . . The kind of flanking attack we're being subjected to now is more difficult to fight off."[25] To complement this piecemeal augmentation of the medical safety net, Democrats began thinking more seriously about ways to craft a contributory, government-based health system for a much broader population. This stood in contrast to the means-tested approach that leading Republicans entertained from the late 1940s forward. However, this tack would allow progressive proponents to argue that this was not simply an extension of welfare, but rather something that workers paid into and from which they would therefore be entitled to draw. The problem with this approach, had it been implemented in the 1950s, was that only about half of Americans over 65 years of age were entitled to Social Security retirement benefits, leaving the other half of them without hospital insurance.[26] However, the proponents of what would become Medicare understood this shortcoming of their plan but also understood that this was the price to be paid to make their strategy a politically viable one.

THE FORAND BILL, KERR-MILLS, AND THE PUSH FOR MEDICARE

In pursuit of the strategy of a quasi-entitlement-based coverage, a group of labor lobbyists and other healthcare advocates drafted a bill that would offer Social Security recipients surgery and nursing home coverage as well as 60 days of hospital insurance. Anticipating resistance along the well-worn track of the socialized medicine argument, the bill included provisions designed to allay fears of a government takeover of medical practices. Under the bill, the secretary of the Department of Health, Education, and Welfare would not be permitted to manage how hospitals administered themselves or how medicine was practiced, nor could the secretary influence the hiring or pay of hospital staff. The bill was to be funded by increasing the portion of wages subject to Social Security taxes.[27] Searching for a sponsor who held a seat on the House Ways and Means Committee, the bill drafters were turned down by Wilbur Mills, the powerful committee chair, and two other members before finally approaching Rhode Island Democrat Aime Forand in 1957.

Forand initially thought the bill's prospects poor, but in time he recognized that organized labor in his home state liked the idea, so he lent his sponsorship. Introduced in August, bill number HR 9467 had a hearing the next year but failed to win committee approval, in part owing to resistance from Wilbur Mills, in addition to opposition by Republicans and conservative southern Democrats. The Eisenhower administration also took a dim view of the Forand bill, with the secretary of Health, Education, and Welfare, Marion Folsom, testifying against it and joining various critics who argued that the bill would cost too much and would intrude on the growing private insurance market.[28] Between 1952 and 1958 the number of people with hospitalization coverage rose from 91 million to 121 million, and the ranks of those enjoying other types of medical insurance doubled from 36 million to 72 million. In light of these trends, according to its critics, the Forand bill seemed to be a solution in search of a problem. Insurance company representatives testified that they opposed the bill because it would dampen the sales of private insurance policies. This, of course, was not a surprising position by insurers, given that during both world wars the insurance industry had opposed government-issued life insurance policies for soldiers.[29]

The leadership of the AMA viewed the Forand bill as "the thin end of the wedge" aimed toward compulsory health insurance and as such a threat to doctors' financial standing and professional autonomy.[30] Despite the 35 percent poverty rate among those over 65 at the time, the AMA leadership, particularly its president, Dr. Edward Annis, insisted that there was no health crisis among the elderly and that there was nothing wrong with that population that the current Social Security program could not address.[31] The AMA hired actor Ronald Reagan to record a speech that made up part of a public education campaign by the Association's Women's Auxiliary. The plan, dubbed Operation Coffee Cup, was to stimulate informal gatherings where doctors' wives socialized and listened to recordings of Reagan's speech, which was designed to motivate people to contact their representatives urging them to kill the Medicare bill. Reagan urged people to

call your friends and tell them to write them. If you don't, this program, I promise you, will pass just as surely as the sun will come up tomorrow. And behind it will come other federal programs that will invade every area of freedom as we have known in this country. Until one day . . . we will awake to find that we have socialism. And if you don't do this, one of these days you and I are going to spend our sunset years telling our children and our children's children what it once was like in America when men were free.[32]

The AMA leadership responded to this renewed push for Medicare by forming the American Medical Political Action Committee in 1958.

Along the way, internal differences complicated the Association's efforts. Some doctors feared that this level of political involvement would endanger the AMA's tax exempt status under the Internal Revenue Code. Others wondered if a scientific association should be so involved in politics. Objections aside, the political action committee was launched in the summer of 1960 with a series of field training sessions to teach physicians about political advocacy.[33] Like the AMA, the American Association of Physicians and Surgeons (AAPS) also opposed the Forand bill. Speaking for its 15,000 members, the AAPS' leadership took the position that if passed this bill "will be such a strong endorsement of the philosophy of Social Security, and will fix so firmly upon the American people the shackles of the welfare state, that most of you . . . will live to see the total and permanent destruction of individual freedom."[34]

Unsuccessful in securing passage in 1958, Representative Forand redrafted the bill, adjusting the tax withholdings and other provisions, and reintroduced it in 1959. He still encountered opposition within his own party, including Wilbur Mills, Sam Rayburn, and even Senator Lyndon Johnson. House Ways and Means Committee hearings provided a venue for various opponents, including the vice speaker of the AMA's House of Delegates who boldly asserted that in his home state of Texas no one went without medical care. In due course, he was forced to concede that charity care provided a significant part of the medical system. His liberal detractors pointed out that charity care and its catch-as-catch-can approach was no way to ensure a continuity of the doctor-patient relationship, purportedly a sacred feature of American medical provision, according to the rhetoric of the AMA over the previous several decades.[35]

In support of the Forand bill, the AFL-CIO argued for its necessity, citing the swelling ranks of the elderly and their increasing difficulty in paying for medical services. According to welfare historian Jill Quadagno, through the latter half of the 1950s the labor organization "became a sort of headquarters . . . for the people who were trying to get something done about health insurance for the aged," organizing printed materials, instructional sessions, networking lunches, and the like, for Medicare supporters.[36] The goal was to reframe the debate into one about the elderly rather than one turning on questions about the overall structure of the economy. The AFL-CIO undertook some communications efforts with its affiliates on behalf of the Forand bill, but those were not much more than routine, as described later by Nelson Cruikshank, director of the AFL-CIO's Social Security department. Organized labor had on its side not only a growing grassroots movement for the bill but also many congressional Democrats.[37] Having gotten on board to support the Forand bill, Senator John Kennedy, along with other senators, toured the country and collected public input from 38 cities during 1959 and 1960. Typical of what the senators heard was a comment from a retired insurance company employee living in St. Petersburg, Florida. "Citizens of this country, over age 65 [who] have worked, saved, and sacrificed, during their productive years to accumulate a home and a few dollars for their old age should not be required to pauperize themselves to get health care."[38] Kennedy insisted at this time that "voluntary health programs have proven that they cannot do the job. Public charity and the generosity of relatives cannot and should not do the job. The [Eisenhower] Administration has shown that it will not do the job. And so a Democratic Congress must do the job."[39]

For his part, Senator Barry Goldwater opposed the bill, claiming that the medical needs of the elderly were not fundamentally different from those of younger Americans, a position that would later cause him some chagrin during his 1964 campaign for the presidency. Goldwater only slowly realized just how low income and high risk—that is, costly to insure—most seniors were at this time. Vice President Nixon found himself in an awkward position in 1960, running for president and realizing that the same arguments used against government-financed medicine in the 1940s and 1950s carried less weight at the turn of a new decade. Nixon attempted to persuade his Republican colleagues to offer their own version of the Forand bill, but Eisenhower initially refused.[40] Finally, in the late spring of 1960 the administration offered a counterproposal involving a complicated tax arrangement and large out-of-pocket expenses, to which critics emerged from seemingly all quarters. Goldwater commented that "it can be dressed up, painted, pictured as voluntary, but any way it is put, the plan . . . for the aid to the aged is socialized medicine."[41] Nixon was so discouraged that he refused to comment. He feared that if the Forand bill passed Eisenhower would veto it, handing the Democrats a ripe campaign issue for the fall. He therefore threw his support to a bill jointly sponsored by Mills and Democratic Senator Robert Kerr of Oklahoma, a bill Nixon believed represented a middle way and one that he hoped would defuse the issue before the November election.[42]

Nixon got his wish. The bill crafted largely by Kerr, who stood for reelection in 1960 and was quite attuned to the cross-pressures facing him, was designed to distinguish the Oklahoma senator from Kennedy and his pro-Medicare position while also not neglecting the needs of a large group of the medically indigent. Kerr feared that if he went all out for the Catholic Kennedy he would "loose a hundred and twenty five thousand Baptists" and that if he came out for health insurance under Social Security, he would "lose every doctor in the state."[43] A middle way offered a better solution. Partnering with Mills, the resulting bill significantly enlarged the federal grants dating back in 1950. States could participate at their option, passing along federally subsidized grants to medical providers who elected to service the poor. Senior advocacy groups did not prefer a charity medicine or means-tested approach. In committee testimony in 1960, representatives from various groups, including the Council for the Aging of Springfield, Massachusetts, and the Los Angeles County Senior Citizens Association, argued that "our senior citizens are independent people. They have a heritage of independence. They do not like to ask for charity. We consider a federal medical-care program the only solution for us on low incomes."[44] The senior citizen organizations did not get their way, but the passage of Kerr-Mills represented another step toward Medicare. The reality was that a means-tested approach met with much less opposition from congressional Republicans than did a more comprehensive, Social Security–based program.

Once it became apparent that Kerr-Mills was going to pass, the AMA switched positions to support the bill, as it preferred this option over the more expansive Medicare proposal. If opponents viewed Kerr-Mills as a stalling tactic, in as much as they saw it as a way to placate moderates who might otherwise throw their support to a more ambitious proposal, supporters of more universal coverage viewed Kerr-Mills as another step taken on what they were increasingly confident was a ladder escalating to something much more broad. Presidential candidate Nixon celebrated the Kerr-Mills bill when it was signed into law but also warned that "the American people . . . do not want, they must not have, a compulsory health insurance plan forced down their throats."[45]

An expanded federal grant program to help meet the medical needs of the elderly and poor fell far short of the compulsory health insurance that conservatives feared, but it certainly represented a step on a ladder. Neither side was completely satisfied with the Kerr-Mills program. Many conservatives viewed it as too much interference in the market, while many liberals worried about the program's reliance on annual appropriations from Congress and buy-in from the states, factors that could seriously limit the program's reach.[46] Democratic Senator Albert Gore, Sr., of Tennessee complained that the new program's means test would erode "the pride of our people to make them go hat in hand to public officials and please their poverty before receiving any aid."[47] Despite this complaint, the step-on-the-ladder argument led most Democrats to support the bill. For their part, some conservatives saw Kerr-Mills as the lesser of two evils, if the Social Security–based Forand bill was the alternative. Given how closely the electorate was divided in 1960, conservatives could probably not have anticipated with clarity the changes that were coming, but within two more congressional election cycles, federal health policy would indeed take two very large steps on the ladder with what would become Medicare and Medicaid. But first, the gradual implementation of Kerr-Mills would impart some useful lessons.

IMPLEMENTING KERR-MILLS AND THE NEXT STEP TOWARD MEDICARE

The enactment of the Kerr-Mills program in 1960 expanded federal subsidies for vendor payments for the elderly, blind, and disabled poor. Most important, it also provided for payments on behalf of persons not receiving public assistance, a break from past policy. Kerr-Mills was to be an open-ended commitment on the part of the federal government. Means tests for eligibility were left to the states, allowing them to decide on their preferred level of generosity. Although federal funds were available by late 1960, many states were slow to adopt this voluntary program. Only 28 had done so by the end of 1962. The early adopters tended to be those that had availed themselves of federal health grants prior to 1960. Because of the state investment required to leverage the federal dollars, wealthier states, for which such investment was easier, tended to utilize the program more aggressively and poorer states less so. Georgia and Mississippi adopted the Kerr-Mills program in 1964, but their legislatures never appropriated any state money for it.[48] Nationwide, only about one-fifth of the hypothetically eligible 10 million Americans enrolled in the program, due in large part to states' reluctance to buy in. Even where they did, the cross-state disparities in investment were almost mind-boggling. Early in the life of Kerr-Mills, New York covered nearly 27,000 individuals, compared to only 571 in Oklahoma. Liberals lambasted the program as "uneven, unfair, [and] undignified."[49]

In time, the creation of this expanded federal grant program helped defuse some of the resistance to government involvement in health care. The medical lobby came to recognize the reality that the availability of government funds to cover healthcare expenses for the medically indigent enabled those services to be paid for as opposed to remaining charity work. One major category of this spending was directed to long-term care for those living in nursing homes. Here, vendor payments grew rapidly in the first few years of Kerr-Mills, from $47 million in 1960 to $449 million in 1965.[50] Further, it became increasingly clear that this government involvement did not spell a loss of professional autonomy. Despite this evolution of thought, old perspectives died hard, and skepticism surrounding government involvement persisted in many quarters. This skepticism was fostered by continued liberal advocacy in Congress for a Medicare bill that would cover a much larger segment of the population than did Kerr-Mills.

The push for Medicare gained momentum with a newly elected president who supported this move. John Kennedy's inauguration prompted the AMA to cite the Medicare proposal as "the most deadly challenge" the Association had ever faced, and it appealed to its 180,000 members to defeat the bill.[51] Pamphlets and posters distributed to doctors for display in their offices warned patients that "Your freedom is at stake. . . . Your freedom to choose the doctor you believe is best for you. And your doctor's freedom— his freedom to treat you in an individual way, adapting his knowledge and skills to your particular problems. These freedoms are bound to be lost when the Federal Government enters the privacy of the examination room— controlling both standards of practice and the choice of practitioner."[52] As the AMA struggled to define its position in these changing times—facing the reality that federal and state involvement had enhanced healthcare fund- ing and trying to welcome that while simultaneously resisting what it saw as encroachments on billing practices and professional autonomy more gener- ally—the leadership of the Association met with in Chicago in late 1961 with William Demougeot. A professor in the speech department at North Texas State University, Demougeot coached them on talking points and pitfalls to avoid. Among other suggestions, he urged them to continue using the "socialized medicine" charge, citing its effectiveness, but to be careful not to use it with "sophisticated people" lest that line of argument come to be seen as hollow. Further, he noted that the charge that the Medicare bill would deprive patients of choice might be powerful, but he cautioned them not to use it with audien- ces that actually knew what was in the Medicare bill because "it simply is not true."[53]

Whether the charge was true or not, the Medicare bill could not quite overcome resistance from Congress members who viewed it as a threat to tra- ditional medicine and government roles. The 1962 fight over the Medicare bill saw a level of intensity probably unseen previously. Although heavily invested in the creation of the Kerr-Mills program, Senator Kerr wanted to draw the line there, and he vigorously opposed further efforts to create a Social Security–based insurance program. He made his private plane available to the AMA to fly opponents of the Medicare bill to Washington, D.C., to pressure members of Congress to defeat the bill. Medical societies across the nation brought pressure to bear on members.[54]

The tide was turning. As 1962 progressed, the AMA leadership took the position that it did not object to public funding for health care for Social Secu- rity recipients so long as the program was administered by a nongovernmental body, such as Blue Cross, instead of the Social Security Administration.[55] Push- ing back while also ceding ground, AMA's pressure was enough to stall the pas- sage of the bill, for the moment. However, the 1962 elections witnessed the reelection of every member of Congress who had supported the Medicare bill. The strength to resist was slowly ebbing out of the nation's largest medical lobby, attributable in part to the changing nature of the debate as the nation's political sensibilities shifted slightly to the left. Furthermore, the percentage of doctors working for institutions on salaries, as opposed to private practice, also sapped the AMA's unity. In the 1920s only about 10 percent of doctors worked for salaries, compared to approximately one-quarter of them by the mid-1950s.[56] Compounding the fracture in the medical profession was the gradual shift on the part of the American Hospital Association from opposition to reluctant support of a Social Security–based Medicare program by 1962. This opened up the possibility for progressive reformers to strike up a new alliance with organized labor and one branch of organized medicine (admittedly, a much less powerful one than the AMA itself) that nudged forward Medicare's prospects, albeit slowly.[57]

When the Medicare bill came up for a Senate vote in 1962, in the form of a rider to a welfare bill that had already passed the House, it failed by a vote of 52 to 48, with 21 southern Democrats and a majority of Republicans against it.[58] This bill would have covered Social Security recipients, regardless of income. Opponents objected that the bill was deficient because it would not accomplish what it sought to achieve, specifically that it would leave an estimated 3 million seniors without coverage because they did not receive Social Security.[59] This must have seemed like a strange argument for the AMA leadership to make, given that its traditional stance had been that even partial coverage of non-needy seniors was too much. In any case, President Kennedy sought to remedy the problem of scope, and in early 1963 he sent up a revised bill that did just that. However, this new Medicare proposal—the King-Anderson bill—also ran into opposition. Insurance lobbyists worked against it, arguing that private insurance coverage among the elderly had expanded from only about 2 percent in 1952 to approximately 60 percent in 1963. There was, therefore, no pressing need for government provision of something the private market seemed able to provide. That argument and related objections prevailed, and when the House Ways and Means Committee considered the King-Anderson bill in 1963 the measure narrowly failed, with 13 votes against and 12 in favor.[60] For proponents, a breakthrough seemed imminent but still just out of reach.

Despite the loss of one of its strongest advocates with Kennedy's assassination, the effort to pass Medicare would remain a prominent piece of work in Congress through 1964. The elections of that year would prove decisive in finally turning the tide. Wilbur Mills understood the implications of the election of many new liberal members to Congress in the fall of 1964 and almost immediately called for new hearings on the Medicare bill within weeks. The most significant change in government involvement in healthcare financing in the nation's history would pass Congress in the summer of 1965 with the creation of Medicare and Medicaid.

NOTES

1. See section 3121 of the Internal Revenue Code.
2. Quadagno 2005, pp. 50–51; Fein 1986, p. 22; Swartz 2006, pp. 45–47; Klein 2003.
3. Quadagno 2005, p. 510.
4. Jecker 1994, pp. 260–263; Quadagno 2005, p. 52.
5. Fein 1986, pp. 22–26.
6. Starr 1982, pp. 295–231; Fein 1986, chapter 2.
7. Stone 1993, p. 301; Harris 1966, pp. 78–80.
8. Jecker 1994, p. 262.
9. Poen 1979, p. 190.
10. Marmor 1999, p. 10; Harris 1966, p. 55.
11. Harris 1966, pp. 55–56.
12. Marmor 1999, p. 15.
13. Altmeyer 1966, p. 202.
14. Ibid., p. 202.
15. Funigiello 2005, p. 91.
16. Quoted in Harris 1966, p. 65; see also Kooijman 1999, p. 144.
17. Harris 1966, pp. 64–65.
18. Ibid., pp. 65–66; Swartz 2006, p. 132.
19. Sundquist 1968, p. 291.
20. Harris 1966, p. 66.
21. Quadagno 2005, p. 45; Poen 1979, pp. 210–211.
22. Quadagno 2005, p. 46; see also Poen 1979, p. 216.
23. Harris 1966, pp. 67–68.
24. Funigiello 2005, p. 89; Poen 1979, pp. 185–186; Altmeyer 1966, pp. 179–189.
25. Poen 1979, p. 213–214.
26. Oberlander 2003, p. 25.
27. Harris 1966, p. 72.
28. Funigiello 2005, pp. 97–98; Oberlander 2003, p. 26.
29. Harris 1966, p. 77.
30. Campion 1984, p. 210.
31. Funigiello 2005, p. 99; Harris 1966, pp. 73–74; see Census Bureau Historical Poverty Tables for 1959 poverty rate (available on line at www.census.gov/hes/www/poverty/histpov/hstpov3.html, table 3, accessed September 11, 2008).
32. Morone 1990, p. 262; see also Harris 1966, p. 139.
33. Campion 1984, pp. 211–213.
34. Harris 1966, p. 82.
35. Funigiello 2005, pp. 100–101.
36. Quadagno 2005, p. 58.
37. Sundquist 1968, pp. 296–299.
38. Ibid., p. 289.
39. Kooijman 1999, p. 144.

40. Funigiello 2005, pp. 101–102; Oberlander 2003, pp. 27–28.

41. "Health Issue Dominates Social Security Debate," *Congressional Quarterly Almanac 1960*, p. 155.

42. Funigiello 2005, p. 103; Fein 1986, p. 57; Harris 1966, p. 114.

43. Harris 1966, p. 111.

44. Ibid., p. 100.

45. Oberlander 2003, p. 28.

46. "Health Issue Dominates Social Security Debate," *Congressional Quarterly Almanac 1960*, p. 148.

47. Funigiello 2005, p. 109.

48. Stevens and Stevens 1974, pp. 30–32.

49. Funigiello 2005, p. 115.

50. Stevens and Stevens 1974, p. 34.

51. Harris 1966, p. 123.

52. Ibid., p 124.

53. Both quotes from Harris 1966, p. 128.

54. Harris 1966, pp. 146–147.

55. Donald Straus, "Criteria for a Good Bill," *The Nation*, 194, #7, February 17, 1962, 134–137.

56. Harris 1966, pp. 149, 76.

57. Kooijman 1999, p. 148.

58. Quadagno 2005, p. 67.

59. Harris 1966, p. 153.

60. Quadagno 2005, p. 67.

4

Enacting Medicare and Medicaid

The 1950s represented a time of incremental policy change, as most advocates for health policy expansion had assumed it would have to be, given the political center of gravity at the time. Conditions simply did not favor bold moves toward significantly greater government roles in health financing or provision. For their part, free-market opponents of government health care enjoyed a triumph following the 1948 defeat of Truman's plan and had, in turn, become more open to conversations about gradual and selective expansions in the areas of hospital and clinic funding and means-tested poverty medicine. As a consequence, this was a time of moderated rhetoric on both sides—though not in all quarters—that, perhaps paradoxically, preceded what would be the largest step toward government health care in the nation's history: the 1965 creation of Medicare and Medicaid.

This chapter details the significant liberal shift in American politics during the early to mid-1960s and how those changes opened the door to momentous steps toward those that progressive reformers had advocated for years. The passage of Medicare and Medicaid extended healthcare access to millions of Americans previously without, and those programs would, in time, become foundations upon which Congress and the states would further build. The creation of Medicare and Medicaid also went a long way toward taking further wind out of the sails of the argument for universal government-organized health insurance. In this latter sense, these two programs provided a significant fraction of a loaf but also reinforced the categorical nature of America's welfare state, offering quite generous benefits to some while leaving others with little.

Several factors contributed to the seismic shift in health policy in the United States during the 1960s. One was the loss of cohesiveness and authority by organized medicine throughout the previous couple of decades, a loss due largely to the tremendous increase in nonphysician professionals in the healthcare field.[1] Another was the growing realization that approximately one out of five Americans continued living in poverty and that more than one-third of those over age 65 were still poor, despite a broad sense of societal affluence. Shocking as this was, the rediscovery of penury, particularly among senior citizens, stoked calls for more assistance for them. Conservatives strenuously and repeatedly argued that recent expansions in private health insurance lessened the need for public programs. Combined with surveys that purported to indicate that large portions of America's elderly were quite happy with their health and their ability to pay for medical services (even though the accuracy of these reports would be hotly contested during the early 1960s), the argument for government health insurance faced an uphill struggle.[2] In 1945 some 32 million Americans had hospital insurance. Impressively, by 1955 that figure had reached about 105 million.[3] But even with this dramatic spread of private insurance, accounts of unmet health needs among the elderly abounded, as they had the lowest rate of private insurance coverage of any age group, still not quite reaching two-thirds as late as 1965.[4]

If opponents of government health care within organized medicine found strength in arguments about spreading private insurance, they also faced challenges within their own profession. Complicating matters for the medical lobby was its own fracturing, as many nonphysicians assumed roles in various allied health professions during the 1950s. By 1960 physicians had become a distinct minority of all health professionals. As of 1965, some 70 percent of physicians belonged to the AMA. However, doctors made up only about one of every four of the nation's health professionals.[5] While the political cohesiveness of medical doctors had never been perfect, by the beginning of this new decade it had lost a substantial measure of the unity it had achieved during the first half of the twentieth century. Finally, Democratic electoral victories in the 1960s, particularly those of 1964, fundamentally altered the ideological tenor of the conversation. With two-to-one Democratic majorities in both chambers of Congress and a liberal Democrat in the White House, Harry Truman's call for universal health care would receive a large down payment in the form of enormously expanded coverage for seniors and the poor. As the former president from Missouri looked on, in the summer of 1965 Lyndon Johnson signed into law a large part of the goal pursued by progressive reformers for decades.

ANOTHER PUSH FOR MEDICARE

Renewed efforts from the 1960 presidential campaigns through those of 1964 focused mostly on the needs of older Americans. Liberal advocates argued that rising health costs saddled the nation's senior citizens with an unsupportable burden and that merely funding hospital and clinic construction or fragmented public health programs would not solve the problem. Further, liberals were generally repulsed by the idea of means testing government medical assistance. For them, this belittled the worth of people who had struggled to carry the nation through the Great Depression and World War II. Opponents of what had by that time been labeled Medicare—usually referencing the King-Anderson bill in particular—repeatedly cited the dramatic increase in the portion of the population covered with some type of private health insurance plan. Further government involvement, they claimed, was unnecessary and would slow what they saw as the inevitability of private arrangements that in time would cover virtually all Americans. Notably, both sides spent most of their efforts discussing the elderly. Given the 1960 passage of the Kerr-Mills program, the focus on seniors took on a new importance for liberal advocates since this was a population that appeared especially deserving and that still lacked sufficient access to services.

In 1964 the medical community divided over the King-Anderson bill, legislation that promised to cover hospital charges for those 65 and older.[6] The AMA opposed it on the basis of high costs and fears of interference with the private medical practice, while the Physicians Committee for Health Care for the Aged through Social Security supported it out of concerns for the welfare of the elderly.[7] Various representatives from the insurance industry testified to Congress that year against the Medicare bill, complaining that the cost would be too high and voicing their resentment toward government interference in the market. However, division emerged even among insurers. Murray Lincoln, president of the Nationwide Insurance Company, supported the bill, in part because it would provide a useful supplement to private insurance already being purchased by the elderly. He believed that not only did the poor deserve help under Kerr-Mills, but the great middle class also needed assistance. Lincoln noted that "I am concerned about the poor, but I am also concerned about the responsible middle-class citizen who has a haunting fear that an expensive illness will wipe out a lifetime accumulation of savings, threaten the ownership of a home or make him submit to the humiliation of a means test."[8] The splintering among opponents hinted at imminent shifts in political alignments on this issue.

Despite signs of progress, the year 1964 turned out to be a frustrating one for Medicare advocates. Several problems stood in the way of getting a bill

through Congress. Serious fights over civil rights legislation complicated matters throughout that spring. Wilbur Mills, the chair of the House Ways and
Means Committee that had jurisdiction over healthcare legislation, strongly
preferred an expansion of Kerr-Mills rather than an entirely new program.
Despite his protests disavowing outright opposition to Medicare, Mills was
a prime obstacle through his way of peppering advocates with technical questions and making requests for cost-benefit analyses, and the like, regarding
their proposals, essentially as a stalling tactic.[9] Further, due to the impending
election, the 1964 congressional session was shaping up to be a short one,
given that members wanted to escape Washington, D.C., in the summer to
attend their parties' nominating conventions and then return to their districts
to campaign for reelection. On top of this came the continuing argument
from the AMA and Senator Barry Goldwater that calls for a government
medical program ignored the steady march of private insurance that had been
progressing for years.[10]

The president, however, disagreed. Lyndon Johnson strongly supported
the King-Anderson bill and spoke about it frequently. Repeatedly during
1964 Johnson rhetorically linked the need to improve the nation's health to
the coverage problems for the elderly. In his January State of the Union
address he began by calling the policy makers to recognize "the health needs
of all our older citizens."[11] Later that month he urged the passage of a "Social
Security health insurance plan" for seniors without means tests.[12] In his
February special message to Congress on health he again emphasized the special needs of the elderly.[13] And so it went all year.

The King-Anderson bill provided for Social Security–based payment for
limited hospitalization. The legislation offered three different coverage
options from which enrollees would select by their 65th birthday. Options
included total coverage for up to 45 days, up to 180 days with patients paying
the first two and one-half days, or up to 90 days with patients paying $10 per
day for the first 9 days. Other areas of coverage included 180 days of skilled
nursing home care, 240 home healthcare visits annually, and care after the
first $20 per month in outpatient diagnostic treatments. Funding for these
services would be covered by a one-quarter percent increase in employers
and employees, a four-tenths percent increase on the self-employed, and an
increase in the income subject to the FICA tax from $4,800 to $5,200.[14]

Passage of this bill in the House of Representatives in 1964 foundered on
opposition from Republicans and conservative, largely Southern, Democrats,
chiefly Wilbur Mills. In a speech on September 28 in Little Rock, Mills laid
out his reasons for opposition. He believed that the level of taxation on wages
for Social Security programs would become onerous if Medicare were enacted
and that these increased payroll taxes would do "serious and lasting damage to

the basic purpose of the [Social Security] program."[15] Mills continued, explaining that the soundness of the Social Security trust funds relied on their conservative principles. He feared that adding a medical benefit would invite escalating costs, beyond incoming revenues, and that matters would be complicated further when recipients, burdened by deductibles, would almost certainly pressure Congress to cover the costs, resulting in runaway expenditures for the program.[16] Mills also harbored concerns about the government role in administration growing too large, preferring instead to see an intermediary there such as Blue Cross. He also believed that those who were already retired should not be covered by the Medicare plan, as they had not contributed to it during their working years.[17] Mills's opposition mattered not only because of his position as chair of the Ways and Means Committee but also because, in the words of political commentators Evans and Novak, he "possessed that rare combination of encyclopedic knowledge of issues, high accomplishment in the art of legislative chicanery, and ideological flexibility that enabled him to change position whenever he pleased."[18] After the clear message of the 1964 elections, that flexibility would be called upon.

In the mean time and despite these objections, passage of the Medicare bill in the Senate prior to the 1964 elections marked a historic moment. This was the first time either chamber had passed a bill embodying a federal responsibility to pay for health coverage for a broad group of citizens. Senate supporters such as Albert Gore, Sr., supported the measure as an alternative to means-tested assistance and because, he believed, it reflected sound insurance principles. Critics, such as Barry Goldwater, dismissed it as foolish. Goldwater put down the Medicare measure because he said that it insulted the intelligence of seniors, extending benefits in kind rather than in cash and that it limited the ability of recipients to direct where their money went.[19] With passage only in the Senate, of course, the Medicare proposal could not move forward.

The failure of the Medicare bill in the House arguably owed less to the resistance of the AMA than had been true in the past. In the wake of incremental expansions of governmental involvement in the 1950s, Americans came to see that such steps could indeed be taken without disastrous consequences. Further, by continuing to fight losing battles, such as medical care for seniors, the AMA had lost some credibility. One particularly interesting moment came in early 1964 when the Surgeon General declared unequivocally that tobacco is linked to various cancers. Strangely, the AMA refused to endorse the Surgeon General's statement and instead seemed to come to the defense of the tobacco industry. The AMA leadership issued a statement that said in part, "long standing social customs and practices are established in the use of tobacco; the economic lives of tobacco growers, processors, and merchants

are intertwined in the industry; and local, state, and the federal governments
are recipients of and dependent upon many millions of dollars of tax revenue."
In response, Democratic Senator Maurine Neuberger noted that she was
not sure if the AMA was riding to the rescue of tobacco producers, but that
she found herself "growing somewhat apprehensive about the concern of the
AMA for the economic well-being of the tobacco industry rather than the
physical well-being of smokers or potential smokers."[20] In a turn of events that
suggested an odd alliance, at almost the same moment as the Surgeon General
issued his statement, the AMA announced it had accepted a $10 million grant
from the tobacco industry to study links between smoking and health problems. These events, as ironic as they may have been, were insufficient to alter
the fundamental resistance in Congress, especially in the House, to an expanded
governmental role in healthcare financing, but they likely contributed to a sense
of the AMA's declining credibility.[21]

The Democrats' inability to enact Medicare was one of President Johnson's
few significant legislative defeats in 1964. Perhaps as a silver lining, this failure handed the Democrats a prominent campaign issue for that season's elections. Health care was among the most significant national issues at the time.
Republican presidential nominee Barry Goldwater, not only having earlier
staked out a position against Medicaid but also calling for the privatization
of Social Security, found himself on the wrong side of this issue, particularly
given that voters identified him more generally with a return to pre–New
Deal social welfare policies at a time when support for liberal programs was
at a high point.[22] White House Press Secretary Bill Moyers advised Johnson
that the Republican nominee's position on Medicare presented "a great
opportunity for us to beat him to death among these older people if we just
play it right."[23] As controversial as Goldwater's position might have been,
positions from his not-too-distant ideological kin prevailed in Congress right
up until the elections of 1964. But change was coming. Against the tide of
liberal Democrats elected that fall, the remaining opposition to Medicare
simply could not stand.

THE 1964 ELECTIONS AS A TIPPING POINT

The electoral landslide that swept Democrats into a position of dominance
opened the way for advocates of Medicare to advance as never before. In 1964
no congressional incumbent who ran and supported Medicare lost.[24] The
electoral outcome boosted the Democratic House majority by 38 seats to
its most lopsided distribution since Roosevelt's landslide of 1936, more
than two-to-one. In the Senate, where Democrats had already held such a
margin prior to the election, the Democratic majority grew by yet one more.

The resounding defeat for conservatives forced them to see that some type of broad government provision of medical coverage for the elderly would soon be a reality. Commenting to reporters the morning after the November elections, long-time opponent Wilbur Mills noted that he would be sympathetic to a Medicare bill. This time, he meant it. In January congressional leaders readily complied with Lyndon Johnson's request to prioritize the Medicare bills, numbering them HR1 and S1, respectively, the first bills given numbers in the 89th Congress.[25] This prioritizing of Medicare fit with findings from private White House polling that found, shortly after the election, that "help for old people" ranked at the top of a list of national policy priorities.[26]

In what proved to be a last-ditch effort to blunt the momentum pent up behind the election outcome, in February 1965 Representative John Byrnes, the ranking minority member on the Ways and Means Committee, offered an alternative to the King-Anderson bill. This more market-oriented approach—dubbed Bettercare—would have coordinated voluntary insurance funded partly by premiums deducted from workers' paychecks, but not from employers themselves, and subsidized by U.S. treasury funds. The voluntary nature of this idea appealed to Republicans, but for Democrats there remained several problems. First, the Bettercare proposal allowed medical providers to assign what they thought were reasonable charges versus set costs, which they saw as an invitation to cost overruns. Because Bettercare was voluntary its reach would fall short of the Democrats' hoped-for universalism. Further, because those enrolling would need to pay part of the premium during retirement, a time in their lives when their income was low, this would create a strain. The bill was more attractive than some previous Republican proposals because of its avoidance of a means test, but it still fell short of garnering any significant Democratic support in the new Congress even though it proposed covering physician bills, as opposed to the Medicare bill that would have covered only part of hospital charges.[27]

Early in 1965 the AMA advanced its own proposal as an alternative to the Medicare bill. The organization's president, Donovan Ward, did not want to bow to the pressure created by the recent elections, noting that as doctors "we do not, by profession, compromise in matters of life and death; nor can we compromise with honor and duty."[28] The AMA's idea, labeled Eldercare, proposed a voluntary plan involving a federal subsidy to private insurance purchases.[29] Whether this was a tactical turn or a mark of desperation, the AMA seemed stubborn, in the opinion of presidential aide Lawrence O'Brien, who commented that "we in the White House were delighted by the AMA's blind opposition to the inevitable."[30] Increasingly confident with the Kerr-Mills program, the AMA also proposed expanding it at an estimated annual cost of $2.1 billion, instead of a new Social Security–based program.[31]

It remained opposed, however, to moving away from a means-tested program. The AMA's campaign for its Eldercare proposal included newspaper, TV, and radio ads and some 10 million pamphlets denouncing the proposed Medicare bill. Its efforts, however, fell flat.

These three proposals—Medicare, Bettercare, and Eldercare—emerged as the major contenders during the spring of 1965. Because all the congressional sponsors of these bills sat on the Ways and Means Committee, the perceived quality of the proposals meant the committee was torn between serious but competing ideas. During a committee session on March 2, the imperative to reconcile these three approaches became clear to Mills. In response, the chairman rather abruptly proposed a merger of them instead of forcing a showdown. In a surprise move, Mills asked if the committee could combine the three into one package instead of picking from among them. This dramatic reversal has been characterized as "one of the monumental turnabouts in U.S. political history."[32] From this stroke of political savvy emerged the famous three-layer cake metaphor: mandatory coverage for hospital services paid for by payroll withholding during one's working years, voluntary physician services paid for by monthly premiums deducted from one's Social Security payments, and a general revenue-funded program for the medically indigent. Stunning though it was to those in the room, this idea enjoyed an immediate appeal among many committee members. The apparent solution also had the effect of taking the wind out of the sails of the AMA; in as much as it included its indigent care program, it gave the Republicans some of what they wanted in a voluntary program, and it gave liberal Democrats the compulsory program they sought. Wilbur Cohen, an assistant secretary in the Department of Health, Education, and Welfare, later noted that "it was the most brilliant legislative move I'd seen in 30 years. The doctors couldn't complain because they had been carping about Medicare's shortcomings and about its being compulsory. And the Republicans couldn't complain, because it was their own idea. In effect, Mills had taken the AMA's ammunition, put it in the Republicans' gun, and blown both of them off the map."[33] Blown off the map or not, Republicans' reservations persisted, and when the committee favorably reported the bill on March 23 the vote fell along party lines. Democrats were jubilant, feeling they could take all the credit for the accomplishment. The 296-page bill, proposing an annual cost of just over $6 billion, reached the House floor on April 8 and passed by a vote of 313 to 115.[34]

Following two weeks of testimony before the Senate Finance Committee, conservative Democratic Senator Russell Long proposed adding a prescription drug benefit and eliminating co-payments. The question as to whether Long's proposal represented little more than a poison pill amendment remained uncertain, but it was narrowly defeated in committee. After three days of debate on the Senate floor, the bill passed by a solid majority of 68 to 21 in early July.[35] The various Senate amendments were mostly dropped in conference, meaning that the efforts by senators such as Long and others to overload the bill by some $7 billion annually were largely unsuccessful. Despite the seeming inevitability of the bill's passage, Republicans remained deeply skeptical. Representative Byrnes, the House Republican spokesperson on the issue, warned just before the final vote, "I still believe the majority is in error, and I think the country will come to regret having pursued this course."[36] Byrnes spoke for many of his fellow partisans, as most Senate Republicans and nearly half of those in the House voted against the bill in the end. After winning final passage (307 to 116 in the House, 70 to 24 in the Senate), President Johnson signed the bill into law on July 30th at the Truman Library in Independence with former-president Harry Truman standing by his side. Johnson said that "no longer will older Americans be denied the healing miracle of modern medicine" and that "no longer will illness crush and destroy the savings that they have so carefully put away over a lifetime so that they might enjoy dignity in their later years."[37] This bill would benefit not only the senior citizens but also the Johnson administration. A July 1964 poll, conducted shortly before passage, found that only 14 percent of respondents thought that the administration was doing a "very good" job "providing medical care for the aged." By August 1965 that figure had risen to 59 percent.[38] Clearly, this was not only a substantively important achievement for the Democrats, but a popular one as well.

The basic provisions of Medicare included 60 days of covered hospital care with a $40 deductible, 30 days of hospital care beyond that with a daily co-payment of $10, 20 days of covered nursing home care, followed by 80 more days at $5 per day, up to 100 home health aide visits following hospitalization, and coverage of 80 percent of the cost of diagnostic tests after a $20 deductible for each series of tests. In order to pay for the program the taxable wage base rose to $6,600 per year, and the tax rate was increased by one-half of 1 percent for both employer and employee. Despite the slight increases in taxation to pay for Medicare, concerns about funding would become a serious problem by 1967.

The emphasis on aid to the aged, which had been a constant refrain from the president and most Democratic members of Congress, meant that the bulk of assistance would occur under the Medicare portion of the law, the newly added Title 18 of the Social Security Act directed at those over age 65. In contrast, Title 19, or the Medicaid portion of the law, emerged instead as a targeted and means-tested program. Medicaid represented a significant expansion, in terms of funding, of the kind of assistance that had been delivered since 1960 under the Kerr-Mills program. Granting states considerable flexibility, Congress permitted them to continue their Kerr-Mills assistance until as late as 1969 if they so desired, or they could drop that and adopt the Medicaid program right away. Because Medicaid (and Kerr-Mills too, for that matter) was voluntary for states, they could also forgo the new program, as several states did for years. Medicaid represented a regularization of federal funding that led directly to better coverage for those who were eligible but did not strive toward universal or even particularly broad coverage. True to the categorical nature of America's welfare state, several classes of people were excluded from Medicaid, including childless, working-age adults, regardless of their income. Future expansions would bring in more parents and more young people, up to age 21, but large swaths of the needy population would not reap any benefits from this new program.

As an extension of Kerr-Mills, many of the contours of Medicaid policy were to be left to the states. Congress indicated in the legislative language that states should fund the program "as far as practicable under the conditions in such state."[39] The language, however, also included some more assertive features. It gave the secretary of the Department of Health, Education, and Welfare the authority to withhold funds from any state not "making efforts in the direction of broadening the scope of the care and services made available under the plan and in the direction of liberalizing the eligibility requirements for medical assistance."[40] Some states made very little effort, even to the point of not adopting the new program at all. Alaska and Arizona adopted Medicaid only years later, relying instead on the Indian Health Service to cover Native Americans who made up large portions of those states' poor populations. Most states, however, saw the new Medicaid program as a reliable, open-ended financial commitment from the federal government, one that provided more than 50 percent of the program's expenditures. Thus within five years nearly all of them adopted it.[41]

The enactment of Medicare and Medicaid represented a great leap forward for liberal advocates. For the first time the federal government had taken on a commitment to fund health services for large swaths of the population and had done so by way of an entitlement arrangement, meaning that the spigot of federal dollars would be exceedingly difficult to close in the future. From another perspective, the enactment of Medicare and Medicaid represented a "useful tactical retreat" from the universalism that progressives had fought for since the early twentieth century.[42] By settling for less and peeling off the elderly, a group that elicits sympathy, this move had the effect of undercutting political support for more bold and far-reaching steps. The logic of targeting the elderly was compelling. Some three-quarters of them lacked health insurance, and approximately 35 percent of them lived below the poverty line.[43] The achievement was significant, but the price paid for this compromise was high in as much as it meant a push for a more comprehensive plan would be shelved for years to come.

IMPLEMENTING MEDICARE AND MEDICAID

Several challenges presented themselves in the 11 months that the U.S. Department of Health, Education, and Welfare had to put Medicare into effect. (They had even less time with Medicaid, since it took effect on January 1, 1966.) An immediate imperative was to enroll eligible seniors in Part B of Medicare, the mandatory component of the program that covers outpatient services. The premium for this part originally stood at $3 per month. In order to achieve actuarial balance, enrolling a large number of seniors as quickly as possible was necessary. This task turned out to be surprisingly successful. Americans over 65 responded well, and most states automatically enrolled seniors who were on state public assistance programs, a move that shifted those beneficiaries from being state charges, regarding outpatient services, to becoming the financial responsibility of the federal government. By the time Medicare was formally launched in July 1966, an impressive 93 percent of eligible seniors were enrolled.[44]

Various other concerns faced federal administrators. Racial discrimination by hospitals provided one such preoccupation. Instead of including a formal civil rights provision that would have explicitly created a robust federal power to enforce nondiscrimination based on race, the law instead allowed the weaker practice of asking hospitals that sought to participate to sign nondiscrimination contracts. Northern Democrats understood that the administration would interpret the law as prohibiting segregation in hospitals, thus they declined to insist on a formal civil rights provision, a move that also allowed Southern members of Congress to tell themselves that local facilities would perhaps be able to continue their segregationist ways.[45] Indeed, many hospitals in the South resisted signing nondiscrimination documents and continued to offer segregated facilities. Of course, this discrimination created problems for would-be recipients who were unable to put their benefits to use at local hospitals, but it also created a politically awkward situation for Medicare administrators. Stubbornly refusing to cooperate, many Southern hospitals either remained outside of Medicare or wrongfully participated in the program despite their continuing discriminatory practices.[46]

One way for noncompliant hospitals to participate was to not sign the nondiscrimination pledge but to seek Medicare reimbursement under the provision that allowed such payments for emergency room visits by Medicare beneficiaries, an exception permitted under federal law. Evidence of almost certainly abusive use of this emergency provision came in a disproportionate number of emergency room claims from southeastern states during 1967. That year, 86 percent of the nation's 21,000 emergency room claims came from the South despite that region being home to a far smaller percentage of the nation's seniors. Mississippi and Alabama alone accounted for 9,400 of them.

By all appearances, hospitals there were billing nonemergency room care under the emergency care loophole.[47] Given this backdoor option, racial integration was not inviting in many communities, compounded by threats of violence directed toward hospitals that entertained such progressive thinking. A hospital administrator in Canton, Mississippi, was visited by four Klansmen who threatened to bomb the hospital if the administrator insisted on integrating rooms. Similar accounts emerged from Alabama.[48] In the face of this situation, President Johnson spoke of the pressing need for broad cooperation. He implored hospital administrators that "you must comply. If you discriminate against some older citizens in your community, you wreck the program for all. The federal government will not retreat from its clear responsibility under the law, and you must not retreat from yours."[49] Proceedings were initiated against a handful of hospitals that did not integrate wards, with the threat of withholding Medicare dollars from the noncompliant facilities.[50]

For a short time, fears of an AMA-organized boycott of the new program worried administrators as well. However, by the autumn of 1965 this concern was laid to rest, as the AMA leadership indicated its willingness to cooperate.[51] Medicare and Medicaid, after all, ensured payment for many patients who were then either charity care cases or who were doing without services due to an inability to pay. Further, despite Lyndon Johnson's personal disgust toward the AMA—in a conversation with AFL-CIO President George Meany, Johnson compared the AMA to chickens lacking the good sense to stop eating even after finding themselves knee-deep in their own feces—his administration went to pains to clarify that no federal agency would dictate patients' choices of physicians and that no federal officer could "exercise any supervision or control over the practice of medicine or the manner in which medical services are provided" under Medicaid or Medicare.[52] It is uncertain as to how far these assurances went toward allaying doctors' concerns, given that as late as 1965 AMA representatives testifying before Congress still insisted that, under Medicare, physicians' decisions would be "restricted by the decisions of untrained government employees" and that the "voluntary relationship between the patient and his doctor" would be eviscerated, turning the nation's seniors into "federal wards."[53] If the president's pleas did little to persuade them, it seems apparent that the promise of more office visits soon being compensated surely had quite a bit to do with the AMA's grudging acceptance of the program.

By 1967 the major early difficulty with Medicare, and to a lesser extent Medicaid, emerged in the form of steeply escalating costs. Initially the annual price of Medicare was estimated at $500 million, above and beyond the premiums paid by recipients. The Johnson administration was content to commit to this new budget line given the importance and popularity of the program.

A year after passage, a poll by Louis Harris and Associates found that 84 percent of respondents thought that the president was doing either an "excellent" or a "pretty good" job handling Medicare.[54] In March 1967 another poll found that 35 percent of respondents wanted to expand Medicare and another 51 percent wanted to keep it as it was. Only 8 percent called for cuts.[55] Popularity aside, however, by this time the steeply rising costs of Medicare—and Medicaid too—were becoming evident. Patients had quickly taken advantage of the services under these new programs, and providers responded with larger facilities and improved technology. Whereas medical costs had risen approximately 7 percent annually from 1950 to 1965, after 1965 hospital prices increased an average of 14 percent per year, a trend that would continue into the mid-1970s. Unfortunately, because of this medical inflation, not even the presence of Medicare reduced the portion of the average elderly person's budget spent on medical care in the decade after Medicare's creation.[56]

From the federal government's perspective the cost of Medicare was particularly shocking. Within its first two years the program had extended coverage to some 20 million people over age 65, or 10 percent of the population, and had paid $8.4 billion in medical bills. By early 1968 it was becoming apparent that the federal government would soon be responsible to pay for more than 20 percent of the nation's healthcare expenditures. Prospective estimates generated in early 1968 placed that figure at 37 percent by 1970. The skyrocketing costs confirmed the worst fears of Medicare critics. Wilbur Mills worried out loud that Medicare was unbalancing the Social Security funding system, and he called the program one of the more serious mistakes of his career.[57] In response to these cost increases, President Johnson urged providers to limit themselves to reasonable charges, but this effort at moral suasion appears to have had little impact.

The financing issues were not limited to Medicare. As an expansion of Kerr-Mills, Medicaid was envisioned as the distinctly junior partner in the 1965 legislation inasmuch as it targeted only the poor. However, within a few years it had effectively turned into an entitlement for a broad range of people with modest incomes. Seeing an opportunity to draw down federal dollars, states initially created generous income limits, which encouraged more people to enroll. Some states aggressively pursued this tactic, with the effect of covering larger portions of their residents but also laying claim to huge federal grants in the process. In 1967 almost half of federal Medicaid grants flowed to New York and California alone. Pennsylvania also designed its program to maximize the inflow of federal dollars. Not all states were so entrepreneurial. Then, as today, the cross-state variation in scope and generosity of services was dramatic. Per capita program costs in 1967 varied from $3.39 in West Virginia to $35.46 in California.[58] Federal administrators were poorly positioned to respond. Staffing of the Medical Services Division in the Department of Health, Education, and Welfare was minimal, precluding rigorous oversight of state plans. As of July 1965 the Division was limited to 23 workers. It soon grew, but not fast enough for the staff to truly scrutinize the many state plans being submitted.[59] As a result of increased physician and hospital charges and grant-seeking state behaviors, by the midpoint of the 1968 fiscal year federal Medicaid expenditures reached $3.54 billion, a burden created by only 37 state programs operational at that time. The administration had projected Medicaid expenditures of $2.25 billion for the entire 1968 fiscal year for 48 states.[60]

Rapidly rising costs catalyzed two lines of conversation. First, efforts at cost containment gained almost immediate traction in Congress. Second, a few proponents of universal health care saw this situation as an opportunity to revisit calls for covering everyone in the hopes of greater uniformity of programming and achieving greater economy of scale. Politically speaking, calls for broader coverage would not produce much, but those for cost control saw considerable activity, both in the states and at the federal level. A chief source of escalating costs was the statutory language permitting government reimbursements for "reasonable costs" and "customary charges" instead of specified prices for particular services. This vagueness in the law meant the federal budget would bear whatever providers asked, and they asked increasingly more as time passed.[61] Complicating matters was the lack of an organizational disposition to challenge medical providers over their billing. Social Security administrators had long cultivated cooperative relationships with providers and planned to continue the same in the interest of smooth implementation for the new programs. As healthcare historian Theodore Marmor noted, aggressive efforts to limit Medicare costs would have undermined this cooperation. Medicare's architects were reluctant to restrain inflation, lest they alienate Medicare providers.[62]

A cautious mood in the Department of Health, Education, and Welfare notwithstanding, various steps and attempted steps through the late 1960s highlighted some changes that would curtail medical spending growth at the margin. Amendments to the Social Security Act in 1967 precluded federal funding of Medicaid to families with income over 133 percent of the federal poverty level. Many states, including California and New York, responded by reducing their eligibility thresholds and the range of services covered.[63] California curtailed its plan to the five core services mandated in the federal Medicaid law: hospital outpatient and inpatient, physician, X-ray, and lab services and nursing home care, in addition to a few other optional services. Outpatient psychiatric services, extended hospital stays, orthotics, and podiatry services would no longer be covered. Similarly, New York reduced its

Medicaid plan in the face of withering criticism from various quarters, including the *Syracuse Post-Standard*, which called the program "insane, fiscal irresponsibility, socialism, New York's Gigantic Giveaway."[64] While perhaps not exactly a giveaway, certainly hospitals faced little incentive to keep down costs. A 1967 study in New York conducted by a dean at the Harvard Medical School found inefficiencies including "wasteful and even harmful duplication of expensive equipment."[65] Beginning the next year, New York's Governor Rockefeller wrung savings from the Medicaid program by tightening eligibility standards, removing some 1 million people from the rolls, or approximately one-sixth of the state's eligible population.[66] Moves to limit federal eligibility for Medicaid to those below the 133 percent of the poverty rate frustrated many in the administration because this meant that people in some states could find themselves eligible for cash welfare payments, implying their inability to purchase the basic necessities but still not eligible for Medicaid. Specifically, in Indiana, families could receive Aid to Families with Dependent Children with income below $271 per month but remain ineligible for Medicaid until their income dropped to $137 per month. In Texas the gap was $39.[67]

Calls for more serious reforms, beyond mere tinkering at the margins, were also part of the Medicaid and Medicare debates during the late 1960s. Senator Russell Long, chair of the Senate Finance Committee, noted in hearings in 1969 that "we want the Medicaid program to provide help to people who need it and we want the Medicare program to look after the medical needs of our senior citizens. We want that care to be of high quality. But, we think it should be provided on a basis that is efficient and economical, not on a basis which is wasteful and extravagant."[68] If federalism meant that states could use their Medicaid programs to draw down funds in creative ways, one solution would be to take away that flexibility. In 1969 the government's Advisory Commission on Intergovernmental Relations proposed a federal takeover of Medicaid in an effort to impose some uniformity on reimbursement levels. This idea met with defeat both at this time and when President Reagan advanced a similar proposal in the early 1980s.[69] Another system-wide effort at cost containment came in the form of mandated hospital utilization review committees that would set boundaries on what duration of stay was medically necessary. The goal was to make charges less arbitrary and more predictable. Some physicians objected to such norming, fearing the imposition of "cookbook medicine" as a result.[70] This fear aside, such efforts were both incomplete—only about 40 percent of hospitals had them in place by 1970—and easily overshadowed by steep rises in per-service and per-day charges. Medicare would soon become an uncontrollable and very large line in the federal budget, but not one easily reduced inasmuch as it served a needy and vulnerable population.[71] From a fiscal perspective, solutions were particularly hard to come by for precisely this reason. Entitlements, once created, are rarely eliminated.

The second significant response to the passage of Medicare and Medicaid was a round of renewed calls for universal coverage. Many advocates proposed this continuing expansion by increments. Supporters of the unsuccessful 1967 congressional legislation that would have added the disabled under Medicare fell into this camp.[72] Social Security Commissioner Robert Ball viewed the enactment of Medicare for the elderly as an important position to solidify in the larger fight for universal coverage. Ball recalled that "although the public record contains some explicit denials [of this intention], we expected Medicare to be a first step toward universal national health insurance."[73] Walter Reuther, of the United Auto Workers, announced in 1968 that he intended to form a committee to consider the idea once more of a comprehensive national health insurance program.[74] In the summer of 1969 the American Hospital Association announced its plan to study national health insurance proposals, and Senator Edward Kennedy called for universal healthcare coverage that December.[75] However, among the trimming of Democratic majorities in Congress, the election of Richard Nixon in 1968, and continuing steep medical inflation, such efforts met stiff resistance and were, of course, unsuccessful.

Looking back on the mid-1960s as a high-water mark for healthcare reform, it must have seemed to supporters of Medicare and Medicaid that the possibilities, while not endless, were expansive. Organized resistance persisted but made little difference in the face of two-to-one Democratic majorities in Congress and a liberal Democrat in the White House. Most important, what did not happen was a shift away from the well-worn American model of governmental financing through private providers. The creation of Medicare and Medicaid did nothing over the long term to displace the growing power of private insurers and for-profit medicine. So long as this model prevailed, extending coverage to all corners of the population would allow only incremental expansion. Segmenting the population into senior citizens, single poor parents of young children, and the like, had the effect of rendering some demographic groups, such as those of working age, seemingly less in need of assistance. This logic, of course, steers policy away from universalism and toward piecemeal arguments about the worthiness of particular groups, terrain that, for better or worse, worked politically for both opponents and supporters of healthcare policy making through the 1960s. It allowed discrete successes while thwarting more comprehensive moves.

For medical providers, the passage of Medicare leveled the playing field between poor seniors and middle-class ones. It led doctors to bill the same amount for any particular service regardless of the income of the patient. This, in turn, put to rest the Robin Hood billing system that had prevailed in years past, one that had involved overcharging patients of means in order to subsidize the charity medicine doctors provided to poorer patients.[76] That point, however, may seem merely academic when compared to the billowing costs of care under these two programs. When a staff report from the Senate Finance Committee declared in February 1970 that "the Medicare and Medicaid programs are in serious financial trouble," its authors likely had no idea of just how expensive those programs would become over the coming years.[77] Medicare would grow to consume ever larger portions of the federal budget, and Medicaid would begin to bleed states of more resources than nearly any other category of program they undertook. Foreseeing this funding crisis, Department of Health, Education, and Welfare Secretary Robert Finch warned in 1969 that "this nation is faced with a breakdown in the delivery of health care unless immediate concerted action is taken by government and the private sector."[78] Unfortunately, Medicaid and Medicare were not designed to easily allow such action, and in fact none of any real consequences was taken during the two decades to come.

NOTES

1. Stevens 1971, p. 425.
2. Feingold 1966.
3. Stevens 1971, p. 426.
4. Engel 2006, p. 4.
5. *Congressional Quarterly Almanac 1965*, p. 236; Stevens 1971, p. 420.
6. The King-Anderson bill was House resolution #3920 and Senate bill #880.
7. *Congressional Quarterly Almanac 1964*, p. 233.
8. Ibid.
9. Funigiello 2005, chapter 5.
10. Feingold 1966, pp. 130–132.
11. Annual message to the Congress on the State of the Union, January 8, 1964 (available online at www.presidency.ucsb.edu; accessed January 16, 2009).
12. Remarks to leaders of organizations concerned with the problems of senior citizens, January 15, 1964 (available online at www.presidency.ucsb.edu; accessed January 16, 2009).
13. Special message to the Congress on the nation's health, February 10, 1964 (available online at www.presidency.ucsb.edu; accessed January 16, 2009).
14. *Congressional Quarterly Almanac 1964*, p. 232; the FICA tax funds Social Security.
15. *Congressional Quarterly Almanac 1964*, pp. 231–232 (quote on p. 232).
16. Ibid., p. 232.

17. Kooijman 1999, p. 156.

18. Ibid., p. 155.

19. *Congressional Quarterly Almanac 1964*, p. 237.

20. Both quotes are from Harris 1966, p. 160.

21. "Why Are Doctors out of Step?" Louis Lasagna, *The New Republic*, vol. 152, #1, February 2, 1965, pp. 13–15.

22. Funigiello 2005, p. 139.

23. Kooijman 1999, p. 163.

24. Sundquist 1968, p. 317; Quadagno 2005, p. 71.

25. *Congressional Quarterly Almanac 1965*, p. 237; Stevens 1971, p. 439; Feingold 1966, p. 137.

26. Jacobs 1993a, p. 192.

27. *Congressional Quarterly Almanac 1965*, p. 238; Funigiello 2005, p. 143; Oberlander 2003, p. 30; Kooijman 1999, p. 165.

28. Sundquist 1968, p. 318.

29. Stevens 1971, p. 439.

30. Kooijman 1999, p. 165.

31. Funigiello 2005, pp. 143–144.

32. Steinmo and Watts 1995, pp. 347–348.

33. Oberlander 2003, pp. 30–31.

34. Funigiello 2005, pp. 145–149.

35. Ibid., pp. 151–152.

36. Sundquist 1968, p. 321.

37. See Sundquist 1968, p. 321, for quotes; see also *Congressional Quarterly Almanac 1965*, p. 238; Funigiello 2005, p. 153; Poen 1979, p. 1.

38. "Please tell me whether you think the Johnson Administration is doing a very good job, a fairly good job, not so good a job, or a poor job on each of these: Providing medical care for the aged." Opinion Research Corporation, July 18–26, 1964 (N = 1,040), and August 2 to September 3, 1965 (N = 1,027).

39. Stevens and Stevens 1974, p. 57.

40. Ibid., p. 67.

41. Engel 2006, p. 51.

42. Fein 1986, p. 54.

43. Ibid., p. 56.

44. Marmor 1999, p. 87.

45. Kooijman 1999, p. 169.

46. Marmor 1999, p. 88.

47. Mal Schechter, "Faith, Hope & Medicare," *The New Republic*, vol. 159, September 7, 1968.

48. Quadagno 2005, p. 91.

49. Funigiello 2005, p. 161.

50. Ibid., p. 162.

51. *Congressional Quarterly Almanac 1965*, p. 238; Marmor 1999, p. 88.

52. Engel 2006, pp. 64–65; see Kooijman 1999, p. 178, for the comparison of the AMA to chickens.

53. Jacobs 1993a, p. 205.

54. "How would you rate the job President Johnson has done in handling Medicare for the aged?" Harris and Associates, August 1966 (N = 1,250 personal interviews).

55. "Besides providing for the military security of the country, the federal government conducts a number of programs in many different areas. I want to run down some of these programs. For each, tell if you think it should be expanded, kept as is, or cut back: Medicare for the aged." Harris and Associates, March 1967 (N = 1,600 personal interviews).

56. Funigiello 2005, pp. 162–163.

57. Ibid., pp. 165–170.

58. Stevens 1971, p. 479.

59. Stevens and Stevens 1974, pp. 78–79.

60. Feder 1977, p. 111; Stevens 1971, p. 477.

61. Marmor 1999, p. 97.

62. Marmor 1999; see also Feder 1977, p. 23.

63. Stevens 1971, p. 480.

64. Engel 2006, pp. 62–63.

65. "Don't Get Sick," *The New Republic*, vol. 159, September 21, 1968, p. 13.

66. W. David Gardner, "Running Out of Money, Not Patients," *The New Republic*, vol. 158, February 17, 1968, p. 19.

67. Engel 2006, p. 51.

68. Stevens 1971, p. 480.

69. Ibid., p. 487.

70. Campion 1984, p. 328.

71. Ibid., p. 328; Feder 1977, chapter 3.

72. Marmor 1999, p. 91.

73. Kooijman 1999, p. 183.

74. Anderson 1985, p. 203.

75. Marmor 1999, p. 92; Funigiello 2005, pp. 172–173.

76. Stevens 1971, p. 451.

77. Campion 1984, p. 327.

78. Stevens 1971, p. 498.

5

Deepening Trouble
with the Healthcare System

The story of the politics of health care in the 1970s and 1980s is largely one of rising costs and the halting and only partially successful efforts to limit the growing burdens on both public and private resources. Skyrocketing expenditures for Medicare and Medicaid throughout the 1970s drove federal and state governments to look for ways to limit the damage. This, combined with the faded enthusiasm for the Great Society programs, made further efforts to expand public programs a distinctly uphill battle. Concerns about costs largely eclipsed conversations about quality and access.

A growing sense that individuals purchase healthcare services much as they buy other consumer goods fostered policy responses that attempted to place limits on consumer demands, responses that largely failed but which set a pattern that would prevail for years to come. One of the key approaches to demand-side cost controls came through the creation of health maintenance organizations (HMOs). These organizations were facilitated by the passage of the 1973 HMO Act. Financial pressures on governments, private plans, and citizens alike made such cost controls attractive, even if the move to HMOs would not address some of the fundamental drivers of inflation in the medical sector.

This chapter traces the political responses to rising costs under Medicare and Medicaid in the early 1970s, the passage of the 1973 HMO Act, half-hearted attempts to create a system of national health insurance under the Carter administration, and the passage and repeal of catastrophic insurance under Medicare in the late 1980s. These episodes set the stage for a protracted national conversation about health financing in the early 1990s, which is

discussed in Chapter 6. Before moving to that period, however, understanding how the funding and access crisis built over a couple of decades is
important. The 1970s and 1980s witnessed many issues rising and falling in
importance, but the most immediate result was the emergence of a widespread
realization that America's healthcare system was badly broken, incapable of
extending coverage to all who needed it, but quite capable of running up
expenses at a rate far beyond what cost-control measures could rein in. If the
1960s represented a time of cautious but optimistic steps toward building a
medical safety net, the 1970s and 1980s surely marked a time of considerable
fraying of it, along with the full blossoming of a sense of pessimism and institutional brokenness.

In response to all this, demand-side cost controls gained prominence during the 1970s and 1980s. In order to understand the efforts at demand-side
cost controls, first understanding the debate over the extent to which healthcare markets work like other markets is vital to grasping the contemporary
debate. Economist Kenneth Arrow's 1963 article offered compelling reasons
to believe that people buy medical services in fundamentally different ways
than they buy other goods or services. Wealthy people do not tend to purchase as many medical services as they can afford, as they often purchase as
large a home or car as they can afford. On the other hand, poor people do
not refrain from consuming needed medical services in direct relation to their
disposable income. Instead, either they obtain the service through public
programs, supported by taxpayers, or they secure it through providers as a
charity, such as from hospital emergency rooms. One should not overstate
this last point. The uninsured do not appear to rely disproportionately on
emergency rooms for noncritical care. In 1997 they accounted for 11 percent
of all nonurgent emergency room visits, and in 2005 they accounted for
16.7 percent of such visits, approximately in line with the proportion of the
population they represent.[1]

Across all levels of income, consumers do not make purchasing choices
based solely on price or notions or personal tastes. In fact, they typically make
purchases based on recommendations from doctors who are often the very
vendors of the services in question. In cases where the goods or services that
are recommended are to be provided by someone else, such as prescription
drugs or specialist services, neither the consumer nor the recommending
physician may know the retail price. The bottom line is that doctors and
patients do not interact in a competitive environment as consumers and producers do in other economic markets. This argument, combined with that of
health care being a basic right of citizenship, composed a compelling call for
government action to extend access to all. Arthur Okun, an economist at
the Brookings Institution, captured the sense of many on the liberal side of

things in the 1970s when he wrote that every American deserved a "right to a decent existence—to some minimum standards of nutrition, health care, and other essentials of life."[2] Policy makers took steps in this direction, though unevenly. A 1985 federal law required hospitals—both public and private—to stabilize seriously ill or injured patients who presented themselves at emergency rooms regardless of their ability to pay.[3]

In a nation wearying of the Great Society programs of the previous decade, this sort of argument drew criticism from free-market advocates and some medical providers, including Dr. George Pickett. Speaking in October 1977, Pickett echoed Ronald Reagan's 1950s' lament of liberties lost to activist government, noting that "rights are hard to live with because we must all yield a degree of freedom to protect them. . . . The right of access to medical care will cost us more than money."[4] Speaking more directly to the argument about healthcare provision differing from other economic markets, the economist Mark Pauly's 1968 commentary as rejoinder to Kenneth Arrow captured some of the themes that would become central to the consumer-driven movement, a movement that led to efforts at demand-side cost controls. Specifically, Pauly noted that insurance, particularly the type without co-payments, created a dilemma wherein no single person faces much of an incentive to curtail his or her use of services, thus costs rise for everyone in that insurance pool. Further, Pauly noted that because people differ in their preferences for medical services, no single insurance plan—especially a one-size, mandated government plan—will achieve efficiency.[5] Note the controversial move on Pauly's part: he assumed that demand for medical care does not exist apart from an individual's preference or taste for it.[6] To make this point explicit, this is to say that the only reason Person A demands more services than Person B (whether they can afford to pay for it is a separate question) is that Person A simply cares more about securing the service. Under this view, one's health condition, ability to recover from illness, or genetic predisposition for disease has nothing to do with the level of services that person seeks. Strongly adopting this perspective implies that consumers should be made to confront strong financial incentives each time they are tempted to seek services and that diverse consumers should not be jumbled into a common pool with others who have quite different preferences for care. Community rating, by this school of thought, is a bad idea.

As for the critique of one-size government insurance, efforts to expand access to basic care paid handsome dividends during the 1960s and 1970s. Substantial improvements were observed in various measures of public health, including a decline in maternal mortality from 68 deaths per 100,000 population in 1953 to 28 deaths in 1969. Life expectancy rose during this period from 67 to 73.5 years. Among children, rates of immunization improved in the late 1960s, particularly for children on Medicaid.

Improvements were seen in the rates of vaccination for diphtheria, pertussis, tetanus, smallpox, polio, and measles. Of course, this came at a cost to the federal and state governments. Medicaid made services more available, and enrollees took advantage of this availability. In California the hospitalization rate among non-Medi-Cal (Medicaid) patients remained essentially stable during the late 1960s while the rate among Medi-Cal patients rose from 217 per 1,000 population in 1968 to 246 in 1970.[7] Despite these overall improvements, by the late 1960s evidence emerged indicating that the United States was not doing well in comparison to other industrialized nations, and cross-group differences stubbornly remained among Americans. By the late 1960s, American infant mortality was worse than in 14 other industrialized nations, and it was nearly twice as high for nonwhite babies as for white babies. Further, life expectancy was some seven years shorter for nonwhites than for whites.[8]

REMAINING GAPS IN THE SAFETY NET

Despite these enormous increases in medical expenditures, by the mid-1970s there still remained large coverage gaps, with some 8 million people—including one-third of the nation's poor—still uncovered by Medicaid as of 1975. The remaining gaps catalyzed liberals to renew calls for universal health care. In July 1970 a newly reformed Committee for National Health Insurance produced a booklet documenting the crisis of rising costs. This committee, headed by the labor leader Leonard Woodcock of the United Auto Workers and noted cardiologist Michael DeBakey, among others, was sympathetic to Senator Edward Kennedy's summer 1970 introduction of a bill to provide universal health insurance via a single-payer system. Neither Kennedy's bill nor a House counterpart made any significant progress that year. Both were reintroduced in 1971.[9]

The gaps in coverage of the poor were aggravated by state and local peculiarities of the Medicaid program, which allowed inappropriate and even bizarre interactions between patients and providers. The case of a gynecologist in rural South Carolina who pressed all his pregnant Medicaid patients to submit to what he called voluntary sterilization and who refused further prenatal care if they declined illustrates how the program's lack of federal supervision permitted abuses. In this case, with the next physician more than 25 miles away and difficult to reach because of a lack of public transport, 67 women, mostly African Americans, submitted to sterilization over a two-year period.[10]

From the perspective of providers, the advent of Medicaid was a mixed blessing. Prior to these programs, doctors performed considerable charity care.

Medicaid now provided partial payment for those services. However, because Medicaid reimbursed at such low rates—often less than the cost of providing the service—and often delayed payment by months, doctors felt that they were taken advantage of. Whereas before they could justify the gratis work as charity care, that justification faded under Medicaid. Given the government's new obligation to pay, providers shifted their expectations, only to be disappointed. As the editors of the *New England Journal of Medicine* wrote in 1967, "the concept of the federal government as a charity case is ridiculous."[11]

From the perspective of recipients, Medicaid was also a mixed experience in the spottiness of its coverage. Individuals who did not fit into one of the narrowly defined categories were simply not eligible, regardless of their poverty or the severity of their medical needs. Between private insurance remaining out of reach and the gaps in Medicaid coverage, the 1970s opened with some 60 percent of families with incomes of under $3,000 lacking health insurance. In response to a growing realization of the gaps, President Nixon's Health Policy Review Group proposed the Family Health Insurance Plan in 1970. The plan not only would have broadened the reach of public programs but also would have built in co-payments and deductibles in an effort to limit expenses. Nixon's plan was estimated to have cost the federal government an additional $3 billion annually, but it would also have significantly reduced the ranks of the uninsured through a combination of government funding and a limited employer mandate to provide coverage for workers at larger firms. Families with incomes between $5,000 and $8,000 annually would have been allowed to buy into the federal system and receive coverage with an annual premium of $300 per person. This proposal was attractive because it would have supplanted the Medicaid programs in the states and all the confusing variations those involved.[12] However, the diminished appetite for more government action to extend health services combined with Nixon's less-than-robust support for his own plan doomed the proposal.

Given the political environment, progress toward universal coverage proved difficult. Advancements in controlling costs, however, would be taken up more seriously in the coming years. The passage of the Professional Standards Review Act of 1970 was among the various efforts. This plan created a regimen to audit medical records, confirming that the services paid for under Medicare were indeed appropriate. Unfortunately, these Professional Standards Review Organizations (PSROs) ended up costing more to operate than they saved the government, according to the Congressional Budget Office.[13] The PSRO system would later be replaced by the Diagnostic Related Groups approach (more on this later). Despite the initial failure of cost controls, this system marked an important departure from Medicare's early days when the federal government paid basically whatever providers charged on a fee-for-service basis, a system that had provided a recipe for fiscal irresponsibility and a general lack of program oversight.

THE HEALTH MAINTENANCE ORGANIZATION ASSISTANCE ACT OF 1973

The most significant response to rising healthcare costs in the early 1970s was the passage of the HMO Assistance Act of 1973. With this modest beginning in the form of grants to support the experimental launch of prepaid health plans, Congress created a legal framework that within 25 years would become the dominant model for private health insurance. Although these ideas were formalized in the early 1970s, the core principles of HMOs had their genesis in the late 1930s. The first modern HMOs appeared in 1938 in Los Angeles when that city needed an aqueduct built. The remoteness of the worksites made medical care for the workers difficult to obtain through community-based physicians. Henry Kaiser, whose construction firm needed to offer medical coverage in order to recruit employees to perform what was at times dangerous work, contracted with a doctor, who was promised a set fee for each employee. Up to this point, and for quite a few years beyond it, employers purchased indemnity-type insurance policies. Employers wearied of the large and sometimes unpredictable expenses associated with indemnity policies and looked for an alternative. Kaiser developed a prepaid plan that assured both that his workers had adequate coverage and that the doctor could enjoy a living under the arrangement. The system worked so well that in 1942 Kaiser created a separate corporation, Kaiser Permanente, to provide coverage for the employees of his shipyard. When in time it appeared that the corporation was going to fail, Kaiser opened enrollment to the public in 1945, and the plan grew rapidly.[14] As of 2009 Kaiser Permanente served 8.6 million people and was still the largest single prepaid, not-for-profit plan in the United States.[15] HMOs were then and are now based on the idea of a prepaid package of services, with agreed fees for each, that cover a group of employees on a per capita basis. Limits apply to the type of services that are available and to the medical providers who sign contracts with the HMOs. They also employ incentives to encourage doctors to practice medicine in a way that the HMO management deems appropriate and profitable.

The more contemporary formulation of HMOs was the brainchild of Minnesota physician Paul Ellwood, who coined the term HMO. He wanted to introduce an improved corporate approach into healthcare financing. Ellwood's original idea was to call these new business entities "health care corporations," but that seemed to carry some "ideological baggage," so Ellwood's study group shifted to the term HMO in 1970.[16] The change in nomenclature, ratified by the HMO Act in 1973, constituted what has been called an act of "premeditated ambiguity."[17] By allowing these new entities to take on a variety of forms, the 1973 legislation permitted private medical practices as well as more traditional insurers to operate as HMOs, making their introduction more appealing to private physicians who otherwise might be concerned about nonphysician business entities taking over the payment management system.[18] This accommodation of private practices under a new financing regime meant that Congress had moved from simply assisting select Americans through subsidies to creating a whole new way for Americans to purchase their health services, a bold move considering the resistance of organized medicine to government involvement over the previous century, and at the time.[19]

The Nixon White House was not a natural locus for sympathetic conversations about further government involvement in healthcare financing. Conservatives in the administration, tired of what they saw as the excesses of the Great Society programs, were inclined toward less, not more, federal involvement in American life. However, Health, Education, and Welfare Secretary Robert Finch and his successor, Elliot Richardson, became key advocates for HMOs. As Health, Education, and Welfare secretary, Richardson had overseen the awarding of over $16 million in federal grants to start-up HMOs in 1970, long before this became a full-fledged item on the White House's agenda or a bill in Congress. A couple of years later, the HMO model provided Nixon an alternative to Senator Kennedy's proposed single-payer system, which the senator was promoting through a series of hearings across the country (while also promoting his potential presidential aspirations). Further, HMOs appealed to conservatives because they were partly market-based, and their initial expansion would be controlled by a Republican administration.[20] In this vein, Nixon also advanced during 1971 his own initiative, the National Health Insurance Partnership, marking the first time since Harry Truman that an American president had called for a national insurance arrangement, albeit based on market mechanisms this time around. When Nixon spoke to the AMA's House of Delegates in June 1971, he pointed out that to put the federal government at the center of coordinating healthcare financing would mean total government domination of health care, not something he wanted to see happen. Kennedy criticized Nixon's overreliance on the private sector. An impasse between contending camps meant that no action was taken prior to the 1972 election.[21] However, the fundamentals of the idea were broadly appealing, and with costs spiraling upward at an alarming rate, the HMO initiative enjoyed considerable support in many quarters.

With the passage of the HMO Act in 1973, some congressional conservatives criticized it as a not-so-sly maneuver toward national health insurance.[22]
The AMA opposed it and sent Nixon's former personal physician, an AMA
executive board member, to talk the president out of his support for it.[23]
Some liberals still wanted to move to a single-payer system. The resulting
compromise was that the federal government would provide, in experimental
fashion, seed money to help launch a limited number of HMOs. The act
authorized $375 million over five years (FYs 1974–78) in the form of loan
guarantees for both nonprofit and for-profit HMOs that were first starting
up and for feasibility studies to help HMOs design their business plans.
Some, such as Republican Senator Robert Taft, argued that a small pilot program would be more appropriate than a multimillion dollar effort, saying
that Congress should adopt a "fly before you buy approach" instead of making such a large investment up front.[24]

In comparison to some other start-ups, this one seemed indeed quite
unambitious. The act's structure effectively limited the number of HMOs
receiving grants to approximately 100. The legislation targeted HMOs
enrolling traditionally under-served populations such as those in inner-city
and rural areas.[25] The stated goals were to increase the number of HMOs
significantly, 250 of them within five years, a far cry from the five to ten thousand initially proposed by the White House. The bill was burdened with the
problems of open enrollment, community-experience instead of individual-
experience rating, and a too-expansive range of benefits mandated.[26] Implementation of the law was delayed due to slow writing of regulations in the
Department of Health, Education, and Welfare. Specifically, the law called
for employers to offer both traditional health insurance and an HMO. Creating administrative rules for this dual-choice provision consumed nearly two
years. Consequently, most large companies delayed in aggressively imple-
menting the HMO option. The restrictions were high enough and the grants
small enough to dissuade many potential organizations from becoming
involved. At the end of its first year of operation, nearly one-half of the appropriated money went unspent due to lack of applicants.[27] Taken together,
these problems resulted in a very slow start for HMOs. By the end of the
1970s only about 5 percent of Americans were enrolled in one.[28]

Despite its modest beginning, the legislative recognition of the contemporary
HMO model represented a significant development. The limited initial impact
eventually gave way to more sweeping propagation of prepaid plans. In the short
term, Congress continued to fund the start-up of HMOs throughout the 1970s,
including $48 million in the fiscal year 1980 budget targeting areas of the coun-
try with the highest healthcare costs. By 1980, 217 plans operated but were generally not seen as much of a political force. The federal legislation legitimizing

them had come to be seen as something of a failure for its inability to propagate them as quickly as some had expected in the early 1970s.[29]

In the longer term HMOs would come to dominate the healthcare market in the 1990s. The crafting of this model overcame what might have been fatal opposition from doctors who, if not for their accommodation under the HMO Act, would have fought this measure of government involvement in organizing payment systems. With its market orientation it won support from fiscal conservatives who otherwise would surely have seen it as yet another step toward a government health insurance program. Corporations, although initially lukewarm toward the idea, appreciated the predictability that HMOs offered, even if neither in the short- nor the long-term they produced dramatic cost savings. Liberals appreciated HMOs because they provided a feasible way to spread employer-based, group coverage to a larger number of workers. In the end, the government endorsement of modern HMOs marked a shift in language, as Paul Starr has written: "The 'socialized medicine' of one era became the corporate reform of the next."[30] This successful blending of a politics of mutual aid with a competition-based formula was a political winner. Looking back on the creation of HMOs in the early 1970s, what might have been initially seen as a minor development in the health system is probably more appropriately thought of as important watershed. As one observer later wrote, the emergence of HMOs marked "a critical juncture in the development of American health care policy, an essential foundation for the subsequent establishment of managed care and managed competition."[31] Their importance lies not only in restructuring how medical services are paid for but also in going a long way toward conditioning the types of services offered. A critical interpretation on this latter point is that HMOs effectively turn doctors into either agents of a corporation intent on minimizing care or liars about the range and type of services that would constitute ideal treatment for a given illness. If HMOs pressure doctors not to provide certain treatments for a given illness, either those doctors are not going to fully inform the HMO about the diagnosis or they will not fully inform the patient about the ways in which treatment is being limited.[32] Either way, the bargain that doctors made during this period gave them a measure of predictability, but in exchange they lost some control over payment amounts and treatment options.

HALTING EFFORTS AT REFORM

Throughout the 1970s and into the 1980s policy makers and the public clearly recognized that medical costs were veering out of control. Despite this situation, serious reform efforts stalled due to continuing ideological conflicts over the role of government and a lack of a clear electoral mandate to act boldly to control costs or extend coverage to the growing millions of Americans without regular access to services. The result was a series of halting efforts during this period. Liberals got part of what they wanted in the form of expanded coverage under Medicaid, particularly for women and children. Conservatives won some minor victories in amendments to Medicare payment rules that fostered market competition. However, the lack of broad solutions meant that piecemeal reform prevailed, addressing cost and access issues at the margins while allowing expenses to mount for public programs and various interests to become more entrenched, thus resistant to future attempts at reform. This was a difficult time for healthcare policy makers, and the failure to address the fundamental flaws in Medicare and Medicaid during their first decade complicated efforts to do so later.

In early 1974, amid the distractions of the unfolding Watergate scandal, the president proposed his Comprehensive Health Insurance bill.[33] In keeping with Nixon's penchant for taking a basically conservative approach to social policy while simultaneously entertaining liberal elements, his plan involved an employer mandate with voluntary participation for employees.[34] Over a three-year phase-in period employers would become responsible for paying 75 percent of the cost of premiums. The administration's bill also called for federally subsidized health care for the poor. The Democratically controlled Congress and the administration appeared to come within compromising distance, but many liberals believed that moving toward the president's plan represented too much of an abandonment of the goal of universal coverage. In April 1974 the Committee on National Health Insurance and the National Council of Senior Citizens, along with other consumer protection groups and organized labor, staked out their opposition to the administration's position. The fight over this bill, of course, was eclipsed by the political meltdown that consumed the summer and by Nixon's resignation in August. By the time a new legislative session began in January 1975, congressional Democrats found themselves facing in Gerald Ford, a president who promised to veto any new federal spending and who instead asked for a tax cut to spur the nation out of a sluggish economic downturn. Bold moves to expand coverage did not seem plausible in this environment of divided government and with a president who lacked an electoral mandate. Ford called for a national health insurance bill, but fragmentation within Congress and tension between the branches thwarted any agreement.[35] Meanwhile, outlays for public programs mounted. By 1975 the share of gross domestic product dedicated to health care in the United States reached 8 percent, exceeding that of all but three nations: Sweden, the Netherlands, and West Germany. Medicaid in particular had risen dramatically due to its much expanded use. Between 1970 and 1976 Medicaid spending increased by 231 percent.[36]

The lack of serious progress of universal health care under the Nixon and Ford administrations also continued under that of Jimmy Carter. Carter proposed the Hospital Cost Containment Act in April 1977. It was designed to help contain costs across Medicare, Medicaid, Blue Cross, private insurance, and private-pay customers.[37] Both chambers of Congress considered the president's bill, but neither passed it. Despite what sympathetically might be called his best effort, Carter was not off the hook with liberals. Senator Kennedy continued his drumbeat for a single-payer system and criticized the president for not doing enough to expand access. When Carter suggested further study of the issue, Kennedy disparaged him for stalling.[38] Caught between competing commitments, Carter apparently saw no ready solutions. On the one hand, he wanted to live up to his campaign commitments to reach universal health care, a promise in which organized labor also held a keen interest. On the other hand he wanted to limit inflation. He saw the need for comprehensive reform, that is, doing more than simply expanding the reach of private insurance; however, he feared running up the federal budget deficit to an even greater extent. At a June 1978 cabinet meeting Carter noted that he wanted to develop a national health policy but that he did not want to substitute public dollars for private ones. He feared inflation, in the form of too many dollars chasing too few goods, by artificially inducing employers to raise wages by the amount they currently paid for private insurance.[39]

Facing pressure from Kennedy on his political left and Russell Long on his right (who had proposed a federally funded catastrophic coverage plan) and backed up against his own 1976 campaign promise to reform the health system, Carter finally proposed a plan in 1979. In an effort of moderation, Carter's National Health Plan would have provided limited government subsidies for payment of private insurance premiums. The president noted at the time that the all-or-nothing approach, referring to Kennedy's bill, had been tried in past years and had failed. Instead, this approach would phase in coverage ensuring that no American would have to pay more than $1,250 annually (government would cover expenses above that). Sixty-six million aged, blind, and disabled persons would be extended coverage without co-payments, an employer mandate would extend help to full-time employees and their dependents, and the federal government would sell health insurance for part-time workers and the unemployed. To the potential relief of states, Carter's bill would also have federalized Medicaid. After much debate in multiple committees and subcommittees, the administration's bill was voted down in November 1979. Subsequently, a compromise bill between the plans of Kennedy and the president passed the Senate in late 1979, but Congress adjourned before that legislation could be sent to the House.[40]

The failure of the Carter plan was certainly not due to any lack of a sense that costs were getting out of control. To illustrate this point, by the end of the 1970s General Motors spent more each year on employee health care than it was paying U.S. Steel for the metal it used to build cars.[41] Instead, the policy-making failure was due in large part to providers' refusal to agree to cost-containment measures. Hospitals in particular resisted the changes proposed in the Carter plan, specifically the idea of regulating the types of services they rendered. However, even the threat of possible legislation led hospitals, beginning in 1978, to voluntarily limit their expenses. For a couple of years that approach showed some progress, but costs again continued their upward march in short order, which in turn prompted another round of legislative proposals beginning in 1981. This pressure was certainly felt by the new Reagan administration, which promptly set about searching for solutions. The most immediate response was to limit eligibility to Aid to Families with Dependent Children, which had the effect of limiting access to Medicaid. Significant cuts were achieved with Reagan's first budget in 1981. Congressional Democrats later reinstated much of the programming for poor people (by adding pregnant women and very young children in 1985 and expanding eligibility for these groups even more in 1988). As research highlighted the link between poor health care and other outcomes, a so-called children's strategy was adopted in the mid-1980s to expand Medicaid to include more kids, even if they were not eligible for Aid to Families with Dependent Children.[42]

Beyond simply cutting budgets, the Reagan administration pursued a couple of policy changes that proved unsuccessful. One was to have the federal government assume complete responsibility for funding the Medicaid program in exchange for the states taking over welfare. This proposed swap failed utterly. The administration could not find a single member of Congress willing to sponsor the proposed legislation, so the idea died without even being introduced into Congress.[43]

Another unsuccessful proposal reflected President Reagan's aversion to further federal regulation of markets. The idea was to give vouchers to Medicare and Medicaid recipients and to encourage them to do as well for themselves as they could do among private providers. That proposal won little support in Congress. As an alternative, the administration turned to a prospective payment system (PPS) for Medicare and Medicaid.[44] This system became law in 1983 and was phased in over four years. It paid hospitals on a prospective basis under what was called diagnostic-related group into which a given patient fits. This contrasts with the previous payment system, under which hospitals were paid for all "reasonable costs."[45] The PPS involved a significant measure of government regulation of hospital billing. Three reasons have been given for this perhaps ironic turn by the Reagan administration toward further regulation of hospitals. First, it became evident to most people that a PPS would produce almost immediate cost savings, whereas a market-based plan would take time to put in place. Second, Richard Schweiker, Reagan's secretary of Health and Human Services, had previously held a seat on the Senate Finance Committee where he worked on PPS plans. Third, the PPS reflected a financial incentive for hospitals to treat patients as efficiently as possible, in a market-like way, if you will. If a hospital could treat a patient less expensively than the plan called for, it could pocket the difference. If the hospital spent more than the plan called for, it had to absorb the loss. This idea of fostering market efficiency appealed to many in the administration.[46] The 1983 adoption of the PPS led to falling reimbursement rates under Medicare and Medicaid relative to private-pay rates and in relation to the actual costs of delivering the service. Table 5.1 compares payments by private insurance to those from Medicare and Medicaid between 1980 and 1990. This changed payment system furthered the shift toward less generous reimbursements under these large public programs, a pattern that would become deeply problematic by the 1990s, but it also helped shore up the funding system for Medicare in particular, at least in the short term. Despite this progress, it should be noted that the PPS does not cover outpatient services. This means that services rendered in doctors' offices and those offered on an outpatient basis in hospitals are not limited by this policy.[47]

The shift away from paying all reasonable costs to paying only those envisioned by the PPS saved money but only in the sense that Medicare and Medicaid costs did not rise through the 1980s as rapidly as they otherwise would have. However, those costs still rose considerably. Similarly, overall healthcare costs continued upward at an alarming rate during the 1980s: nearly 5 percent annually after adjusting for inflation and population growth. This adjusted rate of annual growth exceeded comparable rates in Canada (4.7%), France (2.9%), West Germany (1.7%), and other industrialized nations. This outsized inflation rate came on top of the fact that the United States was already spending significantly more per capita than these nations.[48] There was no slackening in the search for solutions. The funding crisis continued to build.

THE RAND HEALTH INSURANCE EXPERIMENT

The long-running debate over how much price affects utilization of medical services is unlikely to be settled definitively anytime soon. However, a study conducted by researchers at the RAND Corporation between 1976

Table 5.1
Ratio of Payment to Costs for Hospitals under Medicare, Medicaid, and Private-Pay
Patients

Year	Medicare	Medicaid	Private-Pay
1980	0.96	0.91	1.12
1981	0.97	0.93	1.12
1982	0.96	0.91	1.14
1983	0.97	0.92	1.16
1984	0.98	0.88	1.16
1985	1.01	0.90	1.16
1986	1.01	0.88	1.20
1987	0.98	0.83	1.22
1988	0.94	0.80	1.22
1989	0.91	0.76	1.27
1990	0.89	0.80	1.30

Source: Adapted from Oberlander, The Political Life of Medicare (University of Chicago Press, 2003).

and 1981 shed considerable light on the question. The experiment involved approximately 2,000 nonelderly families (under age 62) for four years. The study took place in six areas around the nation and tested the effects of insuring people with plans that involved coinsurance, which enrollees had to pay, at the levels of 25 percent, 50 percent, or 95 percent. Additionally, one plan involved no coinsurance at all, thus offering completely free care. People who would become eligible for Medicare during the study period were excluded because the researchers wanted to be able to control the subjects' medical care costs.[49]

Initially reported in the New England Journal of Medicine in 1981, the study found that when individuals have to pay more for their medical care, they tend to use less of it. At the extreme, people in the 95 percent co-payment group used healthcare services between 25 and 30 percent less than those who received free care. Virtually all types of services, except hospital admissions for children, responded in a similar fashion to the co-payment variation. Across the broad range of subjects in the study, being in the 95 percent co-payment group did not systematically affect health outcomes for the subjects. However, an exception occurred for the 6 percent of study subjects who were both sick and poor. The health of these people was adversely affected by being placed in the high co-payment group. For some ailments, such as tooth decay, serious injuries, and high blood pressure, individuals placed in the free care group ended the study in better condition than when they began. Among those with elevated blood pressure, receiving ample care not only lowered their blood pressure but also reduced their mortality rate by approximately 10 percent compared to those in the high coinsurance category.[50]

In summing up the policy implications of the study, its principal investigator, Joseph Newhouse, wrote that the experiment provided "some support for both free care and initial cost sharing [perspectives]. For most individuals the cost of free care seems substantial and health benefits minimal. As a result, there is a good case for initial cost sharing for the majority of the population. But for the 6 percent of our sample who were both sick and poor, the health benefits of free care were measurable."[51] Newhouse went on to discuss possible exceptions for the sick, the elderly, and the poor, groups that would clearly benefit from readier access to preventative care and early-stage diagnoses that could head off much more expensive treatments—with expenses likely shifted to the rest of us—down the road.[52]

The study's main finding, that for most people free care is costly and not systematically linked to health improvements, was one that was favorably reported in the mass media. The *New York Times* approvingly referenced the RAND study in its 1981 and 1982 editorials. One such piece appearing in January 1982 noted that "when people have to pay even part of the cost themselves . . . they will avoid unnecessary care and seek out cheaper providers," the argument made by the Reagan administration's Richard Schweiker. The editorial concluded that "the Secretary's ideas can advance the cause of cost containment in health care. They deserve serious attention."[53]

Critics pointed out that the RAND study almost certainly underrepresented the poor who are also sick. The finding that this group benefited from free care provided a sound justification for subsidizing care to those who cannot otherwise afford it. When such people obtain care through emergency rooms—a very expensive way of getting it—or so late in the progression of their illnesses that treatments are much more involved, those costs are shifted to others.[54] Further, it is important to note that the relationship between the ability to pay and the consumption of services is still highly imperfect. Being required to cover a 95 percent co-payment did not reduce consumption by 95 percent over the level of consumption seen among the free care group, but rather by less than one-third. Hence, the impact of varying up-front costs works only at the margin, albeit a nontrivial margin. The other side of the argument over price-induced efficiency comes in the form of how payment systems should treat service providers. Using fee-for-service payment arrangements provides an incentive for doctors and hospitals to overserve, though in

the process patients presumably receive very thorough care. Moving to a capitation system, under which doctors and hospitals agree to care for a given
patient for a fixed annual amount, encourages much more efficient treatments,
though that might also involve cutting corners, undertreating, or underdiag-
nosing illnesses. The resulting trade-off led critics of the market model, such
as President Carter's Health, Education, and Welfare Secretary Joseph Califano,
to write in the early 1980s that "the absence of competition, the lack of buyer-
seller tension, and the third-party and fee-for-service reimbursement systems
turn the traditional concept of free enterprise on its head."[55]

Regardless of the question as to how one might view the findings of the
RAND study in hindsight, the strategy of demand-side cost controls gained considerable currency as a result. Systematic figures are not available on this point,
but anecdotal evidence indicates that many employers incorporated the study's
findings into their personnel policies. In 1983 the Xerox Corporation adjusted
upward its employees' co-payments, raising the yearly deductible from $100
per individual and $200 per family to 1 percent of earnings per family. It also
adjusted its coinsurance from 0 to 20 percent. Xerox cited the RAND study
findings in the brochure explaining the changes to its employees.[56]

Even though the healthcare sector provides an imperfect example of a market, policy makers tended to look to cost controls predicated on a market
model. In 1982 Congress passed the Tax Equity and Financial Responsibility
Act, which allowed market competition, in the form of managed care, to be
applied to Medicare patients.[57] On the private sector side, the mid-1980s also
saw the rise of capitation systems. In its full bloom, this would come to be
referred to as managed competition, something the Clinton administration
would unsuccessfully attempt to formalize in the early 1990s. In the mean
time, patchwork reforms would still prevail. To illustrate just how incomplete
and sometimes poorly conceived the reforms of the 1980s were, it is useful to
consider the case of the short-lived catastrophic coverage plan that was
appended to Medicare in 1988 only to be repealed the next year. Comprehensive reforms were still a long way off.

CATASTROPHIC COVERAGE UNDER MEDICARE

Rising costs through the 1980s affected seniors as much as any other
group. Between 1980 and 1985 out-of-pocket expenses for Medicare beneficiaries rose by 49 percent for physician services and by 31 percent for outpatient services.[58] With the president looking for a way to bolster his party's
standing among seniors during an election year, Democrats in Congress still
attempting to expand coverage to fill gaps, and Reagan's new Health and
Human Services Secretary Otis Bowen warm to the idea of eliminating some

of the many coverage limitations built into Medicare, the idea of a catastrophic coverage element gained political traction in an environment that would not have normally fostered it. Brown, a former physician, chaired a 1984 commission recommending the removal of the cap on the number of hospital days Medicare would cover. The commission also recommended eliminating co-payments for hospital and skilled-nursing stays.[59] Bowen's role inside the administration was important in overcoming resistance from the president's Domestic Policy Council, whose leader, Edwin Meese, opposed catastrophic coverage on ideological grounds. Further, private insurance companies interested in selling Medigap plans opposed catastrophic coverage under Medicare, as it threatened their business. However, with Bowen as an advocate in the executive branch and many members of Congress looking for a way to compensate seniors for some of the cuts in Medicare they had recently experienced, the plan passed both houses of Congress by large margins.

The Medicare Catastrophic Coverage Act of 1988 removed the limit on the number of hospital days Medicare would cover and imposed only one hospital co-pay per year, regardless of the number of hospitalizations a person had. Medicare now paid for hospice care for the terminally ill. The effort to add a comprehensive prescription drug coverage at this point, an initiative championed by House Speaker Jim Wright and the AARP, was unsuccessful, though an outpatient drug benefit was added (80% coverage after a $600 deductible). Going beyond this partial drug coverage in the plan would have violated the widespread agreement that this program expansion had to maintain budget neutrality. Social Security taxes had been raised in 1983 to confront looming insolvency, and there was a strong and broad sense that to raise them again so soon would be a political nonstarter. Thus, in what turned out to be a fatal flaw in the plan, Congress took the step of having beneficiaries pay for increases in their own benefits.[60]

Citizen anger boiled over in short order. Specifically, under the new law well-to-do seniors faced increased Medicare premiums (a 15% tax capped at $800 per person), and they were the very group that needed the increased coverage the least, given that they often enjoyed private benefits stemming from prior employment. Under this new plan, 40 percent of recipients paid 82 percent of the expanded program costs.[61] Asking those who needed the benefit the least to pay for most of it meant that, in the words of one informed observer, "a mere five months after passage of the . . . Act . . . senior citizens were in open revolt against the program."[62] Senator John Warner said that "in my 11 years in the U.S. Senate I have never dealt with an issue which has met with such unrelenting opposition."[63] Opposition groups formed around the issue, including the National Committee to Preserve Social

Security and Medicare, Seniors Coalition against the Catastrophic Act, and the National Association of Retired Federal Employees. These groups organized protests that heaped seniors' anger upon members of Congress when they visited their home districts.[64] Part of the anger was attributable to the disproportionate costs falling on upper-income recipients, but another part of it came from popular misunderstandings about the program. A 1989 poll of seniors revealed that only 39 percent of them knew that the plan included an outpatient drug coverage. While only those recipients of higher income would be subject to the add-on premium under the new act, various interest groups published materials that confused seniors into believing that this premium increase applied to all recipients. It was described as "a special tax on senior citizens."[65] Pushing back against this idea of an unjust special tax, even the conservative Senator Alan Simpson, who had voted for the measure, lamented that "the whole United States has been swung on its tail by five percent of their most fortunate cogenarians who don't want to pay for these benefits."[66] Philip Longman wrote in *The New Republic* that "so long as we continue to provide enormous subsidies to the affluent elderly, why shouldn't they help pay for the poor of their generation? . . . The affluent elderly must realize that they may pay a price for their selfishness. The catastrophic fuss has split the elderly lobby and weakened it."[67] Picking up on this theme, NBC's Andrea Mitchell noted that "some say a vocal minority of seniors, coupled with congressional cowardice, have ruined the day for the truly needy."[68] Congress repealed virtually the entire catastrophic care plan in 1989 by large majorities because members simply could not stand the criticism from their relatively privileged constituents. The Bush administration essentially took a walk, saying that it supported the program, but it did not exert any real energy to save it.[69] In an important sense, the passage and rapid repeal of the Medicare catastrophic care plan represented a continuing theme of this period: a crisis mentality regarding cost and access but very little consensus concerning remedies.

PROBLEMS WITH MEDICAID

While consensus was substantially lacking over how to address Medicare's rising costs in this period, the problem with Medicaid was at least as severe, for both federal and state policy makers. During the late 1980s and early 1990s, Medicaid, created in the 1960s as a way to formalize grants to medical providers willing to care for low-income families, came into its own in a highly undesirable way. By the end of the 1980s, after several years of more than 15 percent annual growth in costs, Medicaid had become the second most expensive activity of state governments, right behind funding schools.

Dubbed the Pac-Man of state budgets, Medicaid was gobbling up increasingly large portions of states' fiscal resources, consuming an average of some 17 percent by 1990. From meager beginnings—accounting for only about 6 percent of state spending in the mid-1960s—Medicaid had become a burden that states were willing to do just about anything to control.[70]

Several factors lie behind these increases in Medicaid expenditures, but increasingly expensive long-term care was the primary culprit.[71] Hospital inpatient costs were, between 1988 and 1992, by far the single fastest growing component of Medicaid, increasing at a rate 21 percent above the general inflation rate.[72] A second factor boosting program costs was litigation that forced states to raise their reimbursement rates. The 1980 passage of the Boren Amendment required states to pay hospitals amounts that were reasonable and adequate. Taking advantage of this statutory vagueness, providers sued many states over what the former saw as reimbursement rates that were too low. As of 1991, 29 states had been sued over low reimbursements.[73] Suits typically resolved in courts with states being ordered to reevaluate their payment schedules.[74] It is difficult to estimate how much the Boren Amendment contributed to rising costs, but it concerned federal policy makers enough that it was eventually repealed in 1997.[75] A third factor behind Medicaid cost increases was the federal effort to extend coverage to some of the most vulnerable groups of citizens, such as poor children and pregnant women. Between 1980 and 1991 Congress amended the Medicaid law 13 times, first encouraging and later mandating states to cover the medical expenses of these two groups.[76]

Under this pressure through the late 1980s and early 1990s, states and local providers adopted innovative practices designed to bring some relief. Throughout the 1980s, as reimbursement rates under Medicaid fell, private hospitals found that their Medicaid clientele posed what these hospitals saw as an unbearable burden. The common response was that private hospitals began dumping Medicaid and other uninsured patients onto public hospitals. Because these patients tend to have more complex diagnoses, such as HIV/AIDS, they pose a particular challenge to serve. Between 1981 and 1983, the first two years of the fallout from the budget cuts to various safety net programs, numerous public hospitals reported more than a doubling of the number of annual Medicaid patient transfers from private hospitals.[77] When states passed antidumping laws, they effectively obliged private hospitals to accept Medicaid patients. Physicians' intent on turning a profit protested. Dr. Mohsin Shab in Texas complained about the legitimation of Medicaid and mused that "some Texans must now wonder why they are still buying health insurance" when instead they might get by only with Medicaid coverage. Similarly a Missouri doctor, Ellison Weaver, wrote that "you say that in medicine today there is 'the obligation to serve the poor without pay'. . . . Let me tell you, buddy, I don't do *anything* in this business without financial remuneration."[78] These protests aside, the large amount of free care rendered during the mid-1980s strongly suggests that many, if not most, medical providers saw a moral obligation to care for the uninsured. In 1986 approximately 80 percent of internists working in for-profit facilities provided at least some gratis care.[79]

While providers struggled to confront a tidal wave of Medicaid-related costs, states looked for creative ways to cope as well. In 1986 Congress had created the disproportionate share program, which provided more generous than normal reimbursements to providers working with clientele that was disproportionately enrolled on Medicaid. States soon realized that they could use this program as a grant-getting vehicle. States solicited funds from disproportionate-share providers and then declared those funds as state money invested in their respective Medicaid programs, drawing down larger federal grants as a result. This practice, called bootstrapping, became a cause for protest by the federal Health Care Financing Administration in the mid-1991 and later that year by Congress, which outlawed this procedure under the Medicaid Voluntary Contributions and Provider-Specific Tax amendments.[80]

ON THE VERGE OF REFORM . . . AGAIN?

The story of the debate over healthcare provision and financing during the 1970s and 1980s would be a simpler matter either if it involved a long-running debate over core principles or if some type of far-reaching consensus emerged. Unhappily for would-be reformers, neither of these is the case. The period between the launch of Medicare and Medicaid in the 1960s and the Clinton administration's effort at sweeping reform was instead a time of shifting alliances among traditional versus more progressive-minded physicians, divisions about whether demand-side or supply-side cost controls should be pursued, and disagreements over federal efforts to provide more for seniors at general public expense versus requiring beneficiaries to fund their own program expansions.[81] On at least two occasions, conservatives were the main promoters of greater government involvement—some said intervention—in the medical marketplace. Liberals alternated between satisfaction with partial steps and advancing calls for a single-payer system. The idea that consumers respond in some measure to the price of medical services gained a broad but not quite complete following during this time, and that lent credence to further calls for demand-side controls on expenses. However, on behalf of people of limited means—whether poor families with children on welfare, senior citizens facing staggering hospital bills, or even young professionals facing AIDS—calls for government provision continued, and they met with success in many venues. The one hard truth all observers were able to agree on was that costs were rising out of control and that something needed to be done about that. Beyond this agreement, common ground proved scarce indeed as the 1990s began. For the nation to spend 12 percent of GNP on health care in 1990 and 13 percent by 1992 seemed simply unsustainable.[82]

By the late 1980s managed care had reached a level of penetration in the marketplace that employers and workers alike had become quite familiar with it. In 1988 only 29 percent of those covered by employer-based insurance were enrolled in managed care, but by 1993 that figure had reached 51 percent. Similarly, managed care under Medicaid was undergoing rapid growth during this time as well.[83] As one part of a solution, this seemed like a fairly uncontroversial shift, though protests against the limitations imposed on patients and providers would reach a crescendo by the mid-1990s (more on this in Chapter 7). As the 1990s began there was also a growing but still substantially incomplete sense that health care should be considered a basic right of citizenship. Gravely injured or ill people, with or without insurance, now had a right to be stabilized in hospital emergency rooms. Children in families with income up to 150 percent of the poverty level could be eligible for Medicaid. Pregnant women also enjoyed easier access to that program by the end of the 1980s. Congress had experimented, albeit unsuccessfully, with a prescription drug benefit for seniors. And when Harris Wofford, a Democratic candidate for a U.S. Senate seat from Pennsylvania, ran television ads in 1991 pointing out the irony that prisoners enjoyed free legal counsel while millions of working Americans lacked access to medical services, his come-from-behind victory signaled that perhaps the time was right for a renewed conversation about dramatically improving access. Managed care would provide a takeoff point for that conversation, but so would an effort for governments to manage the sale of private insurance. The blending of public and private was not new. This strategy, after all, was at the center of the Nixon administration's support for HMOs two decades earlier. The struggle for a balance that acknowledges the value of universal coverage while achieving that largely through market mechanisms would not progress as its supporters wished. However, the failure demonstrated once more that the lack of consensus witnessed during the 1970s and 1980s represented something fundamental about American's disagreement—and often disagreeableness—about how to provide people this basic good.

NOTES

1. Emily Walker, "Conventional Wisdom on Uninsured Use of the ED Is Only Half True," report available online at www.medpagetoday.com/EmergencyMedicine/EmergencyMedicine/11402 (accessed July 17, 2009).

2. Engel 2006, p. 131.

3. Budrys 2005, pp. 50, 55; the Combined Budget Reconciliation Act of 1985 took effect in 1986.

4. Engel 2006, p. 132.

5. Pauly 1968.

6. Jost 2007; see also Pauly 1971, Melhado 1998, pp. 225–230, and Buchanan 1968, chapter 4, which was influential on Pauly's thinking. See Fox 1979 for a history of economic thinking on health care.

7. Engel 2006, pp. 107–108.

8. Law 1974, p. 1.

9. Kennedy's bill was S. 4323; Funigiello 2005, pp. 173–174.

10. Engel 2006, p. 124.

11. Ibid., p. 112.

12. Ibid., pp. 114–121.

13. Oberlander 2003, pp. 118–119.

14. For a brief history of Kaiser Permanent, see: http:/xnet.kp.org/newscenter/aboutkp/historyofkp.html; see also Budrys 2005, pp. 120–121; Relman 2007, pp. 71–72.

15. http:/xnet.kp.org/newscenter/aboutkp/fastfacts.html (accessed May 15, 2009).

16. Oliver 2004, p. 706; see Ellwood 1971 and Enthoven 1980 for explanations of this approach.

17. Starr 1976, p. 71.

18. Oliver 2004, p. 706.

19. Starr 1976, p. 66.

20. Falkson 1980, pp. 67–68.

21. Funigiello 2005, pp. 175–179.

22. Public law 93–222.

23. Falkson 1980, p. 84.

24. *Congressional Quarterly Almanac 1973*, pp. 501–502 (quote on p. 502).

25. Ibid., p. 499.

26. Anderson 1985, pp. 212–215 (quote on p. 212).

27. Starr 1976, pp. 74–77.

28. Balkin 2003, pp. 68–69.

29. Falkson 1980, pp. 193–194, 202.

30. Starr 1976, p. 71.

31. Oliver 2004, p. 707.

32. Pellegrino 1997.

33. Nixon's program took the form of bills numbered S 2970 and HR 12684.

34. For a thoughtful treatment of Nixon's ability to appeal to both conservatives and liberals, see Burke and Burke (1974) and their account of his support for welfare reform.

35. Funigiello 2005, pp. 180–185; Steinmo and Watts 1995, p. 354.

36. Engel 2006, pp. 146–148.

37. Anderson 1985, p. 220.

38. Califano 1981, p. 98.

39. Ibid., pp. 109–110.

40. Ibid., pp. 129–151.

41. Ibid., p. 138.

42. Tanenbaum 1995, pp. 937–938; quote on p. 937.

43. Pierson 1996, pp. 163–164; see also Conlan 1998, p. 142.

44. Oberlander 2003, pp. 122–123.

45. U.S. House of Representatives, Committee on Ways and Means 1992, pp. 145–146; see also Oberlander 2003, pp. 120–121; Reagan 1999, p. 22.

46. Oberlander 2003, p. 123.

47. Budrys 2005, p. 49.

48. Holahan et al. 1991, pp. 8–9.

49. Newhouse 1993, pp. 8–9.

50. Ibid., chapter 3 and pp. 338–339.

51. Ibid., p. 351.

52. Ibid., p. 352.

53. Both quotes from "Pay More to Pay Less for Health," editorial in *New York Times*, January 8, 1982, p. A-22.

54. See Jost 2007 for an elaboration of this point.

55. Califano 1981, p. 139.

56. Newhouse 1993, p. 341.

57. Oliver 2004, p. 708.

58. Oberlander 2003, pp. 53–58.

59. Marmor 1999, p. 110.

60. Oberlander 2003, pp. 58–61; Marmor 1999, pp. 111–112.

61. Oberlander 2003, pp. 66–68.

62. Himelfarb 1995, p. 73.

63. Ibid., p. 73.

64. Oberlander 2003, pp. 67–68.

65. Himelfarb 1995, p. 77.

66. Ibid., p. 82.

67. Phillip Longman, "Catastrophic Follies," *The New Republic*, vol. 201 #8, August 21, 1989, pp. 16–18 (quote on p. 18).

68. Himelfarb 1995, p. 84.

69. Ibid., p. 91.

70. *Medicaid Statistics: Program and Financial Statistics, FY 1993*, figure 2, Health Care Financing Administration, Washington, D.C. 1994; Hutchison 1991.

71. Coughlin et al. 1994.

72. Ibid., p. 24.

73. Anderson and Scanlon, 1993; Congressional Research Service 1993, p. 42.

74. Coughlin et al. 1994, p. 104.

75. Holahan et al. 1992.

76. Congressional Research Service 1993, pp. 27–28.

77. Engel 2006, pp. 189–191.

78. Ibid., both quotes on p. 191 (italics in original).

79. Ibid., pp. 191–192.

80. Public Law 102–234; See HCFA notice in the *Federal Register*, August 13, 1993, vol. 58, p. 43184 (Medicaid program: Limitations on aggregate payments to disproportionate share hospitals).

81. Harrington 1975.

82. Relman 2007, p. 43.

83. Oliver 2004, p. 712.

6

The Rise and Fall of the Clinton Plan

If, as the saying goes, politics makes strange bedfellows, discussions over health care in the early 1990s certainly illustrate the point. The unsuccessful effort during 1993 and 1994 by the Clinton administration to advance comprehensive reform stands as a significant near miss that was built on two important competing notions. The first is that healthcare services are subject to market forces similar to other goods or services. This is not a new idea, of course, but as it gained credence between the 1970s and the 1990s it lent force to reformers' efforts to subject how Americans pay for medical care to more direct economic incentives. The second belief is that access to basic health services should be thought of essentially as a right of citizenship. This notion fueled calls from many quarters to strive toward universal coverage, even if proponents of various ideological stripes disagreed widely on just how to accomplish this.

The resulting synthesis of this improbable pairing appeared in the form of managed competition. This concept, developed chiefly by a group of policy thinkers through their annual gatherings in Jackson, Wyoming, was appropriated and retooled by the Clinton administration.[1] The Clinton incarnation of managed competition was to be a form of well-regulated private enterprise (some would say overly regulated) and was designed to wring savings from private insurance arrangements that could then be used to expand coverage to the otherwise uninsured. The blending of market-based mechanisms and the goal of universal access was attractive and enjoyed, according to a good deal of polling, the support of most Americans during the early 1990s. However, uncertainty about possible unintended consequences proved too much for the Clinton White House to overcome. While this attempted public-sector reform ultimately failed, it heralded several private-sector changes that strove toward some similar ends. As ironic as it may seem, some of what the Clinton administration was unable to accomplish through public policy, the private market achieved during the following years. In order to understand this synthesis of ideas, it will be helpful to briefly review each before moving into a discussion of the genesis of the Clinton plan, its experience among members of Congress and the public, and its ultimate failure.

The health-care-as-market viewpoint adopted by conservatives and some moderates during the 1970s and 1980s steered many policy analysts toward thinking about demand-side cost controls, specifically positioning consumers and employers to more directly experience the financial consequences of their decisions. This perspective drew on the RAND study of medical service consumption directed by Joseph Newhouse as well as the published work of economists such as Martin Feldstein and Mark Pauly. Feldstein argued that exempting funds spent on health insurance from federal taxation leads to over-insurance, which in turn leads to consumers using more services than they otherwise would.[2] By directly exposing consumers to a larger portion of the true cost of medical services, they could make more prudent decisions about how much they would use, and the competitive dynamic among service providers would drive down prices as in any other market. Many healthcare economists still embrace this view. For their part, the nation's larger insurance companies warmed to the idea of developing ways to actively manage the risk occurring in their large customer pools instead of simply responding to it with higher premiums. Smaller insurers, on the other hand, were more prone to use experience rating instead of community rating, and thus were more disposed to continue their selective underwriting (critics call this cherry-picking) as a way to minimize risk.[3] The methods of smaller insurers notwithstanding, the idea of managing risk through large-scale pooling of consumers and by leading consumers to more fully appreciate the costs of the services they use continued to foster the growth of HMOs. Applying these principles more broadly under government regulation moves us toward managed competition.

In theory, managed competition would drive down costs and liberate resources that could then be used to expand coverage for the uninsured. The details of just how this would work were sufficiently complex as to not be widely understood or even considered beyond academic circles. At the center of one important group of analysts was Stanford University economist Alain Enthoven. He and the other members of the so-called Jackson Hole Group hoped to use managed competition to head off more intrusive government regulation of healthcare markets. Their plan included an employer mandate to either cover workers or pay into a fund to help subsidize individual purchases of insurance. Under this proposal, tax incentives would encourage employers to purchase the least expensive insurance available in a given market. Expenditures would be tax exempt only up to the price of the least expensive insurance coverage available.[4] The deliberations of the Jackson Hole Group had produced quite a bit of sophisticated thinking over the previous two decades and had attracted the attention and participation of some powerful players, including the AMA, executives of Blue Cross and Blue Shield plans, pharmaceutical industry representatives, and leaders from several major corporations, including General Motors. The problem, however, was that the group faced a publicity problem. They had not yet been able to sell their ideas to policy makers. Help came in the form of the *New York Times*. Jack Rosenthal, who oversaw the paper's editorial page, recognized the deliberations of the Jackson Hole Group as important and deserving of attention. He asked Michael Weinstein, one of his editorial writers, to explore possible ways to address the problems facing the U.S. health system. Weinstein, who attended the February 1992 Jackson Hole gathering, selected the managed competition approach and wrote favorably about it, producing 26 editorials during 1991 and 1992. As this heretofore esoteric set of ideas went mainstream, the rationale for managed competition became more politically viable.[5] Though it would be amended along the way, the idea of managed competition would find its champion in presidential candidate Bill Clinton in 1992.

The controversial part of managed competition came in the extensive reach of the contracts upon which the system is built. Consider HMOs as building blocks. Initially HMOs only governed payment for doctors' services. This meant that once a person entered a hospital as an inpatient, the HMO could become liable for substantially larger payments for services beyond its control. The solution was to develop more extensive contracts with medical providers, including hospitals. As these networks of billing contracts spread, managed competition was born. In time, large corporations with extensive integration would emerge, leading critics to refer to these arrangements not simply as managed competition but rather as managed monopolies. As of 2003 the five largest HMOs—United Health, Wellpoint, Aetna, Anthem, and Cigna—enrolled 68 million people, or 92 percent of all HMO enrollees that year.[6] Whether the Federal Trade Commission can draw and defend a bright line between appropriate merger activity and monopolistic behavior involving restraint of trade still remains an open question.[7]

Beyond a growing belief in markets to bring about efficiency, the other important idea to have gained a serious foothold in this debate is that basic health care should be a right instead of a commodity allocated according to individual resources. An important catalyzing event in 1991 dramatized, especially for Democrats, how politically powerful health care as a political issue can be.

Harris Wofford's 1991 come-from-behind victory in Pennsylvania's U.S. Senate race made clear that efforts to make medical services more widely available could make a successful campaign issue, even if it did not give a clear signal as to how that might be achieved.

The plane crash that killed U.S. Senator John Heinz triggered a special election in Pennsylvania in 1991. Harris Wofford, a former university president with no previous elected political experience, faced a popular former Republican governor, Dick Thornburg. Early in the race, Wofford found himself 44 points behind Thornburg in early polling. In response, he began making the case to audiences that if prisoners had a right to legal counsel, surely law-abiding and hardworking Americans had a right to see a doctor when they are sick. Democratic campaign consultant James Carville believed that only an academic would buy this kind of argument, but the Wofford campaign ran the message in TV ads, and it resonated with voters and the media. Before Wofford's remarkable come-from-behind 10 percentage point victory was in hand, the national media had picked up on the importance of health care as a campaign issue.[8] Wofford's victory was the first Democratic success in a U.S. Senate race in Pennsylvania in 30 years.[9] Certainly, other themes also played important roles in this campaign. However, the heavy loss of jobs and consequently of health insurance during the recession of 1990–1991 seemed to prime the electorate for Wofford's populist message. Further, the Thornburgh campaign appeared tone-deaf regarding the importance of health care as an issue. During the final weeks before the election, Thornburgh's campaign manager, Michelle Davis, complained to the media that her boss's "ideas . . . haven't gotten the spotlight he [Wofford] has gotten with one flimsy issue," and that clear-eyed voters should realize that "Dick Thornburgh is the salvation of this sorry-assed state."[10] These missteps almost certainly reinforced the sense that Pennsylvania voters were hurting and wanted government to pay attention to this important issue.

Retrospective essays on this episode have claimed, for instance, that the Wofford victory "sent an unequivocal message to politicians in Washington about the power of the issue and the need to get a plan in address it."[11] This much is probably true, but what must also be appreciated is that the consensus surrounding health care as a problem did not extend to a similar consensus around solutions. Illustrating this point, *Washington Post* reporter E. J. Dionne referred to it as "the issue from hell"—too complicated to explain and sell to the public.[12] Polls of Pennsylvania voters in 1991 indeed found them divided on policy prescriptions. Just over one-third supported an employer mandate, but 32 percent favored a single-payer system. Wofford voters themselves disagreed on these questions.[13]

A fractured electorate was reflected in a diverse set of approaches taken by national politicians during the early 1990s. Senator John Kerry introduced a single-payer plan in Congress in 1991. Under the Kerry proposal the federal government would have determined a benefits package and a total annual budget for health plans, with states setting physician and hospital fees. Funding would have been provided by a 5 percent payroll tax, a new upper-income tax bracket, and higher taxes on cigarettes and alcohol. Former Senator Paul Tsongas proposed a managed competition plan inspired by the Jackson Hole Group.[14] Situated ideologically between these two, involving more government regulation than the Tsongas plan but less than Kerry's single-payer proposal, Bill Clinton campaigned on and then set to work to develop a managed competition proposal that would consume much of his attention throughout the first two years of his presidency.

THE CLINTON CAMPAIGN FOR COMPREHENSIVE REFORM

In formulating a proposal for comprehensive reform, Bill Clinton worked within several important constraints. The most sweeping option, a single-payer system, was politically uncomfortable for this self-styled new Democrat and would have laid him open to charges from his political Right, including the incumbent President George H. W. Bush who had complained about further government regulation as a stalking horse for proponents of socialized medicine.[15] Clinton himself was determined to achieve reform without asking for new taxes, aside from increased sin taxes, such as those on tobacco. Whatever proposal he adopted had to generate sufficient savings to pay for expansion toward universal coverage. The pay or play idea, which promised to promote an economy of scale and eliminate the cost-shifting problem that occurs when uninsured people obtain services and those costs are passed on to others, appealed strongly to Clinton in late 1991. This, however, did not seem like a politically viable core for his plan, given the reluctance by many congressional Democrats to support it and given the Bush administration's accusations that pay or play represented a slippery slope toward a government takeover of the healthcare market.[16] Clinton wanted to rely on market mechanisms instead of public sector command and control. As a senior advisor later related, Bill Clinton was driven by "a fundamental philosophy that regulation doesn't work, never has, never will. And that it was time to let the market try to work."[17] The result was Clinton's middle-way adoption of managed competition. His election in November 1992 opened the door for him to pursue a bold reform effort.

Within this broad framework, numerous decisions had to be made regarding specifics. In what turned out to be a principal mistake, the president used a very large task force to vet ideas and draft a highly detailed bill that he would eventually submit to Congress in the fall of 1993, a date far beyond his initial pledge to deliver a proposed bill within the first 100 days of his presidency. His choice of his wife to convene the task force placed a highly capable if somewhat strident—some would say inflexible—person at the helm. Together with Ira Magaziner, a business consultant friend of the Clintons who oversaw the day-to-day operations of the group, the president's task force set to work, soon swelling to 630 people as more interests and stakeholders were given places at the table. Paradoxically, the broadly inclusive approach created a sense of entitlement, meaning that those who were not invited to join felt wrongfully excluded. Critics pointed out that the vast majority of task force members were Democrats who generally shared the president's point of view. They also criticized the work of the task force as secretive. Indeed, Hillary Clinton gave no substantive media interviews during the deliberations, staff members were not allowed to talk to the press about the evolving plan, and working papers were not allowed to leave the White House during this time. Three outside groups sued the administration over the matter of closed meetings and argued that federal law stipulates that if a nongovernment employee, such as Hillary Clinton, was permitted to attend, then openness must prevail for others as well.[18] Because its work was substantially complete by May 1993 and owing to the troubles it was causing, the task force disbanded at that point. Dana Priest, the *Washington Post* reporter who covered the story, later commented that the administration "hurt [itself] a lot, because the idea formed that they were creating a 'secret plan.'"[19] The secrecy was in part an effort to provide the task force members with an environment where they could work out the complex and controversial technical provisions of an effective bill. Most important, a guiding principle for the task force was to bring to bear the best possible thinking on how to achieve comprehensive and efficient reforms. President Clinton repeatedly instructed his staff to think about the best ideas rather than to worry about political considerations. He would attempt to handle those difficulties.[20]

Bill Clinton's chief tool in the campaign for reform was his skilled use of rhetoric and an ample supply of flesh-and-blood examples to illustrate the brokenness of the U.S. health system and to tout the remedies promised by his team's deliberations. Using extensive polling to identify concepts and language that would resonate with majority public opinion, Bill Clinton spoke at hundreds of events throughout the spring, summer, and fall of 1993 dwelling heavily on six key themes: security, simplicity, savings, choice, quality, and responsibility. Beyond a barrage of daily faxed messages to interested parties, the president made hundreds of public appearances, including formal speeches, town-hall style gatherings, meetings with journalists and interest groups, and radio addresses. Early polling indicated that the public indeed supported the key elements of the Clinton plan (that support would erode during the early part of 1994), but the passage of time with no bill yet drafted for Congress to consider gave opposition groups ample time to organize against the president. Finally, after more than nine months of work, in November, the president sent his highly detailed bill—stretching over 1,300 pages long—to Congress for consideration.

This lengthy and detailed bill included a handful of provisions that accounted for most of the debate surrounding it.[21] Under this proposal the federal government would organize and regulate the operation of regional health insurance purchasing cooperatives or alliances. A chief idea behind these provisions was to achieve an economy of scale by incorporating millions of subscribers under large plans. The major insurance carriers envisioned that they would play a prominent role here, which led them to essentially stay on the sidelines during this campaign and not actively oppose the Clinton plan. The plan would regulate coverage so as to emphasize basic health services and preventative care, to disallow exclusions based on preexisting conditions, and to enhance portability of coverage as people move between jobs. In order to cover all Americans the proposal built on the employer-based system the country already uses, enhancing that by mandating that employers of a certain size (that size varied throughout this period) purchase health insurance for their workers or pay into a government fund that would then be used to subsidize insurance for the unemployed, the self-employed, and the poor.

In a well-executed effort to explain the rather complex plan to Congress, Hillary Clinton testified in late September 1993 to three House committees and a pair of Senate committees over the course of three days.[22] Her ability to discuss not only the larger vision but also the innumerable details without accompaniment or notes clearly impressed many observers. Perhaps unsure how to attack her message without seeming to attack her personally, most Republicans found themselves handling the First Lady with kid gloves, asking about narrow specifics rather than challenging the underlying premises of the Clinton plan. William Bennett, the former education secretary under George H. W. Bush, complained to reporters after Hillary Clinton's appearance that "in the midst of the largest power grab by the government in recent history, most Republicans are either nowhere to be seen, fawning approvingly, or asking questions about the fine print. Here is a monumental assault on the private sector, on individual liberty, and those sworn to its defense are largely silent."[23] Newt Gingrich, then the assistant majority leader in the House, noted after the testimony that "if Ira Magaziner had tried to defend that same plan, he would have been destroyed" and that it was merely good manners that led the Republicans to give the First Lady such a friendly forum.[24]

The chivalry, if that is what it was, quickly wore off. Within a few weeks opponents were lining up to criticize the Clinton plan, some with proposals of their own, others simply determined to deprive Bill Clinton and the Democrats of a victory that threatened to cement Democratic allegiances for years to come. On the theme of legacy building and partisan advantage, the conservative commentator William Kristol wrote a widely read strategy memo in early December that argued that Republicans should strive to "kill," not merely amend, the Clinton bill. Kristol wrote that passage "will re-legitimize middle-class dependence for 'security' on government spending and regulation. It will revive the reputation of the party that spends and regulates, the Democrats, as the generous protector of middle-class interests. And it will at the same time strike a punishing blow against Republican claims to defend the middle class by restraining government."[25] On policy grounds alone, in addition to partisan considerations, Kristol urged his fellow Republicans to "erase" rather than amend the Clinton plan and to emphasize that America's healthcare situation is not in crisis, that the sky is not falling, and that market mechanisms can achieve the necessary fine tuning.

Congressional Republicans adopted a strategy substantially in line with Kristol's advice, though many of them did not want to be seen as being outright obstructionist. Throughout the autumn and into the winter, Republican Senator Bob Dole publicly promised not to play the role of, in his words, "Dr. Gridlock," but he did very little to broker a compromise of any sort.[26] Newt Gingrich, on the other hand, was more straightforward. Appearing on *Meet the Press*, he called the Clinton plan a "monstrosity," a "disaster," and "the most destructively big government approach ever proposed."[27]

Kristol and Gingrich had company in their effort to sow doubt in the public's mind about the Clinton plan. Despite the president's heavy rhetorical reliance on the ideas of "security for all" and "health care that can never be taken away," the Health Insurance Association of America (HIAA), which mainly represented small to mid-sized insurance companies, had begun running a series of television spots in early September that featured a typical middle-class couple named Harry and Louise sitting at their kitchen table, pondering and vocalizing the disconcerting uncertainties of the president's plan.[28] The ad campaign proved highly effective over the next several months. The tone of Harry and Louise's conversations was one of skepticism without presenting any alternatives to the Clinton plan, and they gave no acknowledgement of the trade-offs between the costs of the president's proposed changes versus the savings and improvements to be achieved. The ads often ended with the refrain that there has to be a better way of reform than what the president had proposed. Positioning itself out front via the Harry and Louise ads, the HIAA came to be seen as the administration's chief foe, even though it was, in fact, one of many, but one that severely irritated the president and his allies.

In November the administration's fight with the HIAA became very public when Hillary Clinton, in a speech to pediatricians in Washington, D.C., berated insurance companies for standing on the wrong side of things. She took them to task for "being able to exclude people from coverage, because the more they can exclude, the more money they can make." Responding directly to the Harry and Louise ads, Mrs. Clinton continued, saying that "they have the gall to run TV ads [saying] that there is a better way, the very industry that has brought us to the brink of bankruptcy because of the way they have financed health care."[29] The unintended effect was that over the succeeding weeks newspapers and television stations enlarged the life of the story, giving even more publicity to the HIAA and extending the reach of the Harry and Louise ads far beyond what the association itself could afford to spend. The ads became a common reference point for media conversations about the president's plan, something that numerous critics were beginning to label as overly ambitious.[30] This, in turn, triggered more donations to the insurance lobby, enriching an ad campaign that originally planned to spend only $4 million with more than $15 million in short order.[31] These funds, of course, were augmented by the $1.9 million spent by the AMA's political action committee during 1993 and 1994.[32] The president knew that he had picked a difficult target, but he only later came to appreciate just how thorny it would be to challenge an industry that accounted for approximately one-seventh of the nation's economy, an industry that had many hundreds of millions of dollars at stake each year.[33]

One might wonder why the administration proposed a liberal package of reforms and later displayed a willingness to move somewhat toward the political center as needed rather than to put forth a more moderate bill in the first place. The answer lay in the realization that many Democratic members of Congress supported a single-payer system and would have felt completely abandoned by the president had he positioned his bill in a more market-based way than he did. Persuading these liberals that such a moderate proposal would have been the best they could expect was thought to be a non-starter, politically speaking. For instance, Representative John Dingell, Jr. was determined to lead an effort in the House for a government-based system. He had introduced his own such bill every year since arriving in Congress in 1955. In this perennial crusade, he was carrying on the work of his father, John Dingell, Sr., an early proponent of universal coverage.[34] President Clinton acknowledged this deep commitment on the part of many liberals, but he also believed that once negotiations were joined and the need to move to the center became clear, his fellow Democrats would come along without much trouble.[35] Hillary Clinton later wrote in a memoir that the idea of government-managed competition presented itself as one that could unite a fragmented Democratic caucus in Congress, a political strength, while also enhancing the overall system efficiency.[36]

As negotiations over the sprawling bill proceeded throughout the winter, public support for the president's plan gradually declined. Some 60 percent of the public had approved of the Clinton plan in September, but by late January 1994 that figure had fallen to approximately 50 percent. Some observers attributed the decline in support to distractions and troubles the administration faced on other fronts during the summer and fall, such as the death of Hillary Clinton's father, the suicide of White House aide Vince Foster, the disastrous failure of a military mission in Somalia involving the death of 18 U.S. service members, problems with a U.S. peacekeeping mission in Haiti, an attempted coup against Russia's President Boris Yeltsin, and intensifying Palestinian-Israeli peace negotiations.[37] While these setbacks may have revealed Bill Clinton's limitations and consumed much of his time and energy, they were not associated with a significantly declining job approval rating during this period. Instead, the decline in public support for the Clinton plan seems to have been attributable directly to unfavorable public and elite discourse on the plan itself. The relentless raising of concerns over unintended consequences, negative perceptions of the enlarged government bureaucracy that the plan would require (something like 90 new commissions or agencies, according to estimates), and the nagging issues of cost to the tax payers and the possible loss of choice as to one's medical providers and the procedures they might, or might not, be allowed to prescribe eroded support. The general public seemed to be slipping beyond the reach of Clinton's rhetoric. In response, the White House shifted its strategy beginning in early 1994 to target politicians and opinion leaders. From that point forward, instead of most of the president's carefully engineered rhetoric being directed at the general public, some 60 percent of it was now aimed at political elites, according to an analysis by Lawrence Jacobs and Robert Shapiro.[38]

While it is easy in retrospect to see that this shift in strategy was ineffective, it seemed at the time like a promising move, or at minimum the least-bad option for a White House staff increasingly beleaguered by criticisms from many sides and few allies willing to speak forcefully for the president's carefully tailored proposal. Some observers have pointed to this middle part of the campaign for comprehensive reform and have argued that while the Clinton administration possessed a good sense of the most effective public rhetoric needed to sell its ideas to the public, it had a less clear grasp on how to build a political coalition around those ideas. Slow to send a concrete proposal to Congress, the Clinton White House provided ample time for its opposition to organize. Further, President Clinton's staff was halting in its efforts to build an alliance with potential supporters, specifically with the multimillion member American Association of Retired Persons (AARP). In 1994 the AARP finally threw its support behind the principles of the Clinton plan, but that endorsement, belated as it was, proved far less effective than it might have been had it come earlier.[39] Perhaps part of the difficulty rested with the AARP itself. The negative experience related to its endorsement in 1988 of the Medicare catastrophic insurance legislation, a misstep that cost it dearly among many of its more affluent seniors, had perhaps instilled a measure of caution in its leadership. Perceptible doubts among seniors over what the Clinton plan might involve for them almost certainly inhibited the AARP from jumping into this monumental fight with both feet at an early date. Whatever the reason, the lack of a broad alliance behind the Clinton plan made it more vulnerable than perhaps it would have otherwise been. When critics found their voices in the autumn, the president's prospects quickly grew dim.

CRITICISM AND ALTERNATIVES

At the beginning of 1994, the White House renewed its push on the president's bill. However, by this time critics had fully developed their own arguments against it, and several alternative plans had emerged in Congress. Republicans on the far right had long staked out positions of absolute unwillingness to use the president's bill as a starting point for negotiations. For example, an essay by Representatives Dick Armey and Newt Gingrich appearing in the *National Review* in February 1994 argued that under the Clinton plan "all Americans will have to rely on the government for health care, and the government will tell them what they can get, where they can get it, whom they can get it from, and how much they can spend for it. If you like the way the Federal Government runs public housing and the state government runs the Department of Motor Vehicles, you'll love health care under the Clinton Plan."[40] As a portrayal of the president's bill, this summary exaggerated a good deal, but by this point truthfulness mattered less than the artful manipulation of political symbols and fear-mongering. That same month, perhaps the premier piece of opposition rhetoric appeared in *The New Republic*. Penned by Elizabeth McCaughey, a fellow at the conservative Manhattan Institute, this essay elaborated the ways in which the Clinton plan would purportedly deprive Americans of choice and would inhibit healthcare providers in their freedom to practice medicine as they see fit. McCaughey indicated that she had read the entire 1,342-page bill, and she heavily peppered her sweepingly critical and considerably biased essay with page citations, giving her the impression of being a consummate truth-teller (this from the same commentator who in 2009 would inaccurately but forcefully characterize a House bill as requiring seniors on

Medicare to consult with panels designed to promote hastening the end of life.[41] The essay lambasted price controls as mechanisms that would surely force doctors to give up private practice and to sign on with devious and autonomy-crushing HMOs. Health maintenance organizations, in McCaughey's view, represented much of what was wrong with efforts to control markets, as they strongly coerce or even compel doctors to withhold certain types of procedures in the interest of cost savings, often embargoing significant portions of member-doctors' annual payments until the end of the year in order to ascertain that those doctors have been playing by the HMO's rules. To hear McCaughey tell the story, the Clinton plan's emphasis on basic, primary care imposed inappropriate limits on advanced or specialized care. For those with special needs, this was a disaster. She ominously stated that "another cost-cutting measure in the Clinton bill deprives people over 65 [on Medicare] of access to new cures" because of the federal government's ability to blacklist companies that do not conform to efforts to reduce costs.[42] In the end, according to McCaughey, "the Clinton plan will prevent people from buying the medical care they need . . . [and that] . . . price controls on new drugs will keep people over 65 from getting the medications that can help them. Most important, government controls on medical education will limit what future doctors know, costing lives and suffering no one can calculate."[43] A fierce indictment indeed.

Long-time health policy analyst Theodore Marmor would later respond (in 1995) with his own article in *The New Republic* calling McCaughey's article a "particularly good example of distorted analysis, comparing an idealized past with an unrecognizable caricature of President Clinton's reform bill."[44] He went on to say that McCaughey's article "misrepresented American medicine as unobtrusive fee-for-service care, a system that has largely vanished."[45] Of course, by that time the curtain was drawn on the Clinton plan, and the damage was done.

Undermining the effort to advance Clinton's sweeping reforms was the inability of the administration to sell the idea of managed competition as a market-based solution to control costs. Despite the administration's attempts to represent this idea as an effort to blend government-orchestrated cost-control efforts and market mechanisms, critics persisted in seeing this as simply more government regulation. An angry exchange between Hillary Clinton and Ralph Johnson, the CEO of Johnson and Johnson, captured this crucial disconnect: Johnson wondered out loud, "you've said that these regional alliances that you're thinking about aren't regulatory bodies, but as I hear what Mr. Magaziner says, they're going to collect premiums from employers, they're going to negotiate with providers, they're going to set standards for employer participants in their alliances, they're going to cap rates. They sound like regulatory agencies to me." Hillary Clinton slammed her fist on the table and insisted that "I said they were purchasing cooperatives, and that's what they're going to be!"[46] John Ong, present at the meeting in his role as the chair of the Business Roundtable, understood at that moment that Hillary Clinton was not being particularly open-minded about this matter.

Plainly, the administration's difficulties with conservatives were numerous. To a lesser extent it also faced some challenges from disaffected liberals. Beyond the matter of not advancing a single-payer system, others on the Left also took exception to the idea of limiting choice under government price controls. David Himmelstein, Sidney Wolfe, and Steffie Woolhandler captured some of these criticisms in their hard-hitting essay in the *American Prospect* in the spring of 1993, just before Clinton launched his plan. They argued that managed competition was essentially a corporate welfare approach to the problem of cost because of the way it would privilege large insurers when forming the health insurance purchasing cooperatives. Further, they insisted that "managed competition has never worked anywhere," and that it represents little more than an aggressive elaboration of the government support for HMOs begun under the 1973 HMO Act.[47] They also feared that due to the extensive administrative support required by HMOs—to review charges, proposed services, and the like—that these new supersized HMOs would experience so much overhead cost that they could not possibly save money. Compounding the problems, managed competition would surely limit consumer choice, particularly among those who could not afford comprehensive plans. The partial convergence of criticisms from both sides illustrated just how complicated it would be to assemble a workable alliance to advance meaningful reform.

The resulting fragmentation posed a serious difficulty for the supporters of the Clinton plan. Competing proposals siphoned off would-be supporters and had the effect of complicating the comparison among plans as they proliferated. Within the president's own party, Tennessee Representative Jim Cooper offered a proposal that was also based on the work of the Jackson Hole Group. As a fiscal conservative, however, Cooper did not include an employer mandate in his bill. Instead, he relied on limits on insurance company premiums and taxation of the value of deluxe health plans. Although Cooper succeeded in securing Senate sponsorship by Louisianan John Breaux, his proposal to tax the value of health benefit packages irritated many constituents within the Democratic Party, including organized labor, which considered (at that time and still) good quality health plans as hard-won prizes from corporate management over the past several decades.[48]

As the months progressed, particularly once it became clearer during the late spring and early summer of 1994 that the Clinton plan was not likely to succeed, numerous other plans emerged. Beyond the Cooper plan, alternatives that garnered significant conversation included plans by Missouri Democrat Dick Gephardt, Maine Democrat George Mitchell, Rhode Island Republican John Chafee, and Kansas Republican Bob Dole. Shifting coalitions formed and reformed around these proposals throughout the summer, but in the end the contentious matter of funding, specifically the employer mandate, proved to be too difficult to resolve. Bill sponsors also struggled to define just how close to universal coverage their bills would come. Unsubstantiated claims abounded, and extensive arguments broke out not only over the desirability of attempting certain policies but also over the issue of whether those proposals would achieve what they promised.

THE DEATH OF THE CLINTON PLAN IN CONGRESS

By late June 1994, signs were increasingly clear that the White House proposal that so many people had worked to draft and had hoped to push through Congress' legislative labyrinth simply could not garner sufficient support. During the last week of June, Representative John Dingell, Jr. notified House Speaker Foley that he could not muster enough votes to pass a bill out of his House Energy and Commerce Committee.[49] Attempts continued through late August to fashion a compromise—Senate Majority Leader George Mitchell's so-called Mainstream Coalition was one of them—but the efforts proved unable to overcome the complexity of the issues involved and the fights over how to fund such a bold endeavor in an era of soaring budget deficits. On September 26, Senator Mitchell pronounced the end of the campaign for broad healthcare reform legislation.[50]

Opponents were gleeful. Texas Senator Phil Gramm celebrated, saying "I think America rejoices that the President's health care plan is dead. This is American democracy at its best." Haley Barbour, chair of the Republican National Committee, told the media that "we find ourselves in this position because the Clinton administration proposed creation of a government-run health care system. The more people learned about Clintoncare, the less they liked it."[51] Senator Bob Packwood commented to his Republican colleagues upon achieving the defeat, "we've killed health care reform. Now we've got to make sure our fingerprints are not on it."[52] For his part, President Clinton initially said nothing publicly about the defeat. Instead, his office issued a press release saying in part "I am very sorry that this means Congress isn't going to reform health care this year. . . . But we are not giving up on our mission to cover every American and to control health care costs. This journey is far, far from over. For the sake of those who touched us during this great journey, we are going to keep up the fight and we will prevail."[53] The president and his allies would not prevail, at least not in the short term.

ASSIGNING BLAME: HOW COULD SO MUCH COME TO SO LITTLE?

The postmortems had begun before the formal announcements came from congressional leaders. In time, several explanations for the defeat of reform emerged, including several book-length treatments.[54] This episode would also renew the very long debate among political scientists over the foundational issue behind why America is the only industrialized country lacking national health insurance.[55] On this point, while surely there are institutional factors that help explain the failure (it is the fault of our system and its multiple veto points), attitudinal factors also certainly played a role (Americans are conflicted about whether basic health care ought to be a right). Regarding this particular campaign for reform, several schools of thought emerged regarding where blame might be placed. For shorthand we might refer to them as follows: it was Bill Clinton's fault for incompetently handling the political campaign; it was the public's fault for not knowing what it wanted; and lastly, our institutions are to blame for not lending themselves to simple majority rule. These perspectives are treated in turn over the next few pages.

It Was Bill Clinton's Fault

Overreach is a word used by many to describe the primary flaw with the Clinton administration's plan to advance reform. Republicans and moderate Democrats felt like they had no place at the table and that from the outset Clinton's task force was stacked with people intent on creating a new government regulatory scheme that simply did not square with their ideas of how private markets ought to be the heart of America's healthcare service delivery system.[56] When critics cited the lengthy page count of the White House bill, the charge was implicit or explicit that the administration planned to micromanage healthcare delivery, violating, among other notions, the long-standing idea of the doctor-patient relationship. Corralling Americans into large purchasing alliances, regulating prices for private insurance policies, and requiring employers to provide insurance for their workers all represented too much of a break from what people had been doing for years. Small businesses disliked the employer mandate. Small to midsize insurance companies disliked the purchasing alliances. Medical providers worried about the influence of the insurance companies on the type of services they might offer. What the administration was attempting to achieve alienated too many stakeholder groups in too many ways. Whereas change in the healthcare policy—and most other areas too, for that matter—had typically been governed by incrementalism, this legislation proposed some dramatic breaks at a time when most Americans distrusted government to handle routine matters, much less to oversee a remaking of a sector that represented approximately one-seventh of the U.S. economy.

Whether the administration's greater willingness to compromise would have overcome the objections to the bill is a question that misses at least two important points. First, tackling the funding problem in piecemeal fashion in the mid-1990s would likely not (and will not, going forward) have been a promising solution. The strength of the administration's bill relied on the interconnectedness of its parts. Even the president's own team members acknowledged the difficulty of selling this much complexity to a skeptical public. Paul Starr, a member of the Clinton's inner circle on health care, later wrote of the plan that "there were too many parts, too many new ideas, even for many policy experts to keep straight."[57] That said, the president's plan was complex because the problems to be solved are complex. Many of the president's opponents refused to directly acknowledge this point. Terry Hill, spokesman for the National Federation of Independent Businesses, an anti-Clinton group, commented in September 1994 that "the biggest thing [that led to the downfall] would be the reluctance of the administration to go for anything but the whole package. . . . They refused to try to get incremental reform, and it was either their package or nothing."[58] Incrementalism in American politics carries with it a powerful if perverse logic: it is the way most policy change occurs, but it precludes certain types of highly useful solutions, akin to the reason why people the world over persist in using QWERTY keyboards, even though other layouts enhance typing speed dramatically.[59]

The second point missed by asking about a greater willingness to compromise has to do with House Republicans. Led by Newt Gingrich and Dick Armey, a large number of House Republicans were intent on depriving President Clinton and Democrats more broadly of a political victory that might have relegated the Republican Party to years in the political wilderness.[60] Gingrich, who opposed serious conversations with the Clinton White House from the beginning on this issue, finally showed his true colors on the night of the 1994 election that gave his party control of both chambers of Congress, announcing that Bill Clinton and the Democrats are "the enemies of normal Americans."[61] With this kind of opposition, to seek compromise is to pursue a fool's errand.

Paul Starr commented on the effort, noting that "we had a historic opportunity, and we blew it."[62] Might a different strategy have led to success? Perhaps, but the Monday-morning quarterbacks who found it easy to criticize the Clinton administration's approach need to bear in mind that American politicians have been trying since the nineteen-teens to reform how we pay for health care, with little success. It is, fundamentally, a very difficult task.

It Was the Public's Fault

Some observers instead turned their criticism toward the public. Harvard University's expert on public opinion on health matters, Robert Blendon, was prominently of this position. Blendon believed that the public was profoundly uncertain about what it wanted in the way of reform and that in a time of little confidence in government the flood of complex and difficult to understand ideas about reform left ordinary citizens vulnerable to strong countervailing messages from the administration's critics, including not only opposition partisans in Congress but also the insurance companies and lobbying groups.[63] Blendon cites exit polls from Pennsylvania during the 1991 Wofford victory showing that the public was deeply divided. Keystone State voters were nearly as supportive of a single-payer system (32%) as they were of an employer-based system (35%). Wofford's own voters were similarly split.[64] It seems that when competing plans were offered simultaneously, public support for each fell significantly, suggesting that the public had a very hard time making up its mind.

As voters struggled to make up their minds, they continued sending legislators at least three key messages in the early to mid-1990s: they were worried about the rising costs of health care, they wanted government action but did not specify what that action should be, and they were concerned that the solution could be more harmful than the present illness.[65] By 1994 polling evidence was fairly clear that the majority public (57%) worried that the Clinton bill would run up healthcare costs even more than they already were, and 29 percent were concerned that universal coverage would not be achieved.[66] By this view, the public did not give its representatives clear, usable signals upon which to act, even though it was telling those officials that something needed to be done.

Blendon was not alone in taking this perspective. Josh Wiener of the Brookings Institution adopted a similar position. In Weiner's view "Americans are schizophrenic about health care. They believe that the U.S. health care system needs major reform, but they are quite content with their own health care. . . . Americans want the problems fixed without making major changes in the way their own health care is financed and delivered. But the problem cannot be fixed without significantly changing the way health care is financed and delivered."[67] Part of this criticism seems to hinge on the insight that people often embrace their own suboptimal situations to the exclusion of solutions that require some change but improve matters over the long term. Fear of the unknown plays a major role in inhibiting new learning.

Why the public finds itself in this weak position presents a puzzle. Space limitations do not allow that to be fully elaborated here, but briefly, one solution points back to elected officials themselves. Observers such as Theda

Skocpol believed that rather than an incoherent public being to blame, arguments among elites and opinion leaders sent the public so many conflicting messages that the resulting public confusion was practically expected.[68] Criticisms of the public-at-fault line of argument point bear some consideration. First, the power of organized pressure groups and the money they funnel to members of Congress should never be underestimated. The few hundred million dollars spent by opposition groups, particularly but not exclusively by the National Insurance Association of America, had no counterpart that could speak to the need to reform a wildly inefficient healthcare financing system. In the end, policy failure perhaps should be laid at the doorstep of interest groups, not at that of the general public.[69]

Complicating matters is the proposition that Americans hold quite tightly to an attitude of individualism, not, in the words of Joseph White of the Brookings Institution, to "an ideology of solidarity."[70] White reflects on the idea "that a majority supports the goal of universal health insurance is irrelevant. Majorities also desire a balanced budget, would like to eliminate the Castro regime, and so on. The question is whether majorities support means to attractive ends and whether those means are in fact plausible" in light of the individualistic ethos so widely, if selectively, embraced by Americans.[71]

A variation on this response frames this episode as a case of enduring class conflict. Because the United States lacks a robust and organized working-class identity, political struggles play out not in popular electoral terms but rather as interest group conflict. One exponent of this perspective, Vicente Navarro, writes that "this is why the corporate class and its instruments in the United States oppose establishing government-guaranteed universal entitlements: They strengthen the working class and weaken the capitalist class. The staggering power of the capitalist class and enormous weakness of the working class explains why health care reform failed again."[72]

Our Institutions Are to Blame

Finally, a third line of explanation points not to uncharitable political actors or a weak public but rather to our political institutions and their fragmentation. While certainly designed to foster protracted deliberation and to act as a brake on hasty policy making, our elaborate system of checks and balances also provides organized interests so many places to stop reform that it makes passage of national health insurance "impossible," according to this perspective.[73] Beyond bicameralism and the traditional tensions inherent in interbranch politics, the Clinton plan was subjected to primary jurisdiction in five congressional committees and partial jurisdiction in seven others.[74] Our weak parties cannot effectively serve as conduits for electoral pressure to catalyze major reforms in the face of a fragmented political environment. Overcoming this problem is not simply a matter of mobilizing large numbers of people with the desired policy preferences. The multiple veto points hard-wired into our system perpetually leave the door open for yet another organized interest to muddy the waters.

*   *   *   *

Regardless of whose fault it was, the public conversation about managed care quickly disappeared within a year of the failure of the Clinton plan. The trend line in Figure 6.1 shows the number of newspaper stories containing both the terms "managed competition" and "health" appearing in a sampling of newspapers, by calendar quarter, from 1990 through 1995 (see figure notes for details). Virtually unheard of until the third quarter of 1991, the term managed competition rose in use at first slowly and unevenly but then

Figure 6.1
Number of Mentions of "Managed Competition" in Print Media, 1990–1995

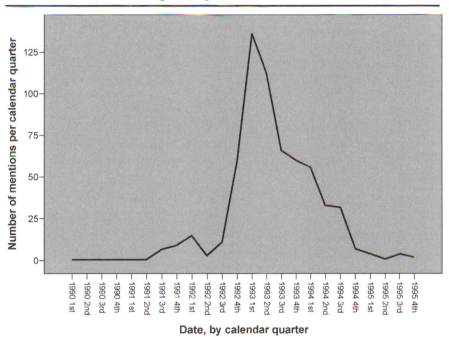

Source: Computations by author based on electronic searches of mentions of "managed competition" and "health" in nine newspapers and the Associated Press via the Lexis-Nexis news archive (*Atlanta Journal and Constitution, Christian Science Monitor, Boston Globe, Chicago Sun-Times, Denver Post, New York Times, Philadelphia Inquirer*). Counts were tabulated by calender quarter from the beginning of 1990 through the end of 1995.

steeply through the first half of 1993, only to fall as steeply thereafter and to virtually disappear from public view by the middle of 1995. This idea, developed so systematically by the Jackson Hole Group and then modified by the Clintons, went from obscure, to commonplace, to politically rejected over a four-year period.

In light of the mighty but failing struggle to pass sweeping health reform and the alienation that had caused among voters, President Clinton's pollster Stan Greenburg advised Democrats in a long memo written in the early fall of 1994 that they should stay away from health care while out campaigning for reelection. "Talk about something else," Greenburg urged them.[75] It was time to move on.

NOTES

1. See Ellwood and Enthoven 1995 for a brief explanation of the Jackson Hole Group plan.
2. Feldstein 1973; see also Melhado 1998.
3. See Hacker 1997, chapter 2 for discussion.
4. Skocpol 1996, pp. 42–43.
5. Hacker 1997, pp. 63–66; Oliver 2004, pp. 710–711.
6. Budrys 2005, pp. 123–124.
7. See Federal Trade Commission 2004 and Hyman and Kovacic 2004.
8. Skocpol 1996, pp. 25–30.
9. Johnson and Broder 1996, p. 60.
10. Quoted in Dale Russakoff, "Thornburgh's 44-Point Lead Vanishes," *Washington Post*, October 31, 1991, p. A-1; and Michael deCourcy Hinds, "Democrats Look to the Senate Race in Pennsylvania for Lessons and Hope," *New York Times*, October 23, 1991, p. A-14, respectively.
11. Oliver 2004, p. 710; see also Hacker 1997, chapter 1.
12. Starr 1992, p. 11.
13. Brodie and Blendon 1995, p. 405.
14. Johnson and Broder 1996, pp. 71–73.
15. Jacobs and Shapiro 2000, p. 81.
16. Skocpol 1996, pp. 34–39.
17. Jacobs and Shapiro 2000, p. 79.
18. H. Clinton 2003, pp. 153–154; J. Jennings Moss, "Clinton Prescription Rejected by Body Politic," *Washington Times*, September 22, 1994, p. A-10.
19. Johnson and Broder 1996, p. 142.
20. Adam Clymer, Robert Pear, and Robin Toner, "The Health Care Debate," *New York Times*, August 29, 1994, p. A-1; Jacobs and Shapiro 2000, chapter 3.
21. See White House Domestic Policy Council 1993 for a full account of the Clinton plan.

22. H. Clinton 2003, pp. 188–189.

23. Adam Clymer, "The Clinton Health Plan Is Alive on Arrival," *New York Times*, October 3, 1993, section 4, p. 3.

24. Ibid.

25. Kristol memo, available online at http:/www.scribd.com/doc/12926608/William-Kristols-1993-Memo-Defeating-President-Clintons-Health-Care-Proposal?autodown=pdf; accessed May 22, 2009; see also Johnson and Broder 1996, p. 234.

26. Quoted in Jacobs and Shapiro 2000, p. 137; see also Robin Toner, "The Health Care Debate: . . . " *New York Times*, September 27, 1994, p. A-1.

27. Jacobs and Shapiro 2000, p. 137.

28. Ibid., p. 134.

29. Johnson and Broder 1996, pp. 209–210.

30. Jacobs and Shapiro 2000, p. 138.

31. Johnson and Broder 1996, p. 212.

32. Steinmo and Watts 1995, p. 364.

33. Ibid., p. 363.

34. David Rosenbaum, "The Health Care Debate: Behind the Scenes," *New York Times*, July 2, 1994, p. A-7.

35. Johnson and Broder 1996, pp. 300–306.

36. H. Clinton 2003, p. 150.

37. Ibid., pp. 182–184; Jacobs and Shapiro 2000, p. 235.

38. Jacobs and Shapiro 2000, pp. 140–142.

39. Skocpol 1996, p. 93; see also Robert Pear, "Clinton Fails to Get Endorsement of Elderly Group on Health Plan," *New York Times*, February 24, 1994, p. A-1.

40. Dick Armey and Newt Gingrich, "The Welfarization of Health Care," *National Review*, February 7, 1994, p. 53.

41. Paul West, "GOP Rides Wave of Ire," *The Baltimore Sun*, August 16, 2009, p. 1-A.

42. McCaughey 1994, p. 25.

43. Ibid.

44. Marmor 1995, p. 500.

45. Ibid.

46. Johnson and Broder 1996, p. 319.

47. Himmelstein et al. 1993, p. 116.

48. Johnson and Broder 1996, p. 313.

49. David Rosenbaum, "The Health Care Debate: Behind the Scenes," *New York Times*, July 2, 1994, p. A-7.

50. *New York Times*, "Health Reform—Dead for Now," September 27, 1994, p. A-24.

51. Both quotes from Johnson and Broder 1996, p. 528.

52. Johnson and Broder 1996, p. 521; Robin Toner, "The Health Care Debate: . . . " *New York Times*, September 27, 1994, p. A-1.

53. Johnson and Broder 1996, p. 529.

54. Skocpol 1996; Hacker 1997; Navarro 1994.

55. See Steinmo and Watts 1995, and Quadagno 2005.

56. Robin Toner, "Pollsters Say Health Care Helped Sweep away Democrats," *New York Times*, September 16, 1994, p. A-14; "The Health Care Debate: In Their Own Words," *New York Times*, September 27, 1994, p. B-11.

57. Starr 1995, p. 23.

58. Quoted in J. Jennings Moss, "The Story So Far," *Washington Times*, September 13, 1994, p. E-1.

59. Diamond 1997, p. 248.

60. Jacobs and Shapiro 2000, chapter 4.

61. Peter Applebome, "Nation Joins South as Its Traditional Politics Gain Favor," *The Atlanta Journal and Constitution*, November 24, 1994, p. F-10.

62. Starr 1995, p. 21.

63. Blendon quoted in J. Jennings Moss, "The Story So Far," *Washington Times*, September 13, 1994, p. E-1.

64. Brodie and Blendon 1995, p. 405.

65. Brodie and Blendon 1995.

66. Ibid., p. 406.

67. Skocpol 1996, p. 12.

68. Ibid., p. 13.

69. Jacobs and Shapiro 1995.

70. White 1995, p. 376.

71. Ibid., p. 379.

72. Navarro 1995, p. 458.

73. Steinmo and Watts 1995, p. 329.

74. Funigiello 2005, p. 301.

75. Johnson and Broder 1996, p. 516.

7

One Piece at a Time?

Moving beyond the failure of the Clinton plan meant attempting a series of small steps to address important access and cost issues that persisted. This was particularly true owing to the highly contentious nature of divided government during the remainder of the 1990s. A highly polarized Congress and acrimonious interbranch relations complicated matters when it came to solving these complex problems. Small steps characterized this period.

This chapter traces these attempts—some successful, some not—including legislation to enhance the portability of health insurance for those who have it, fights over patients' rights in the face of HMOs intent on limiting expenses, challenges to Medicare based on a consumer-driven logic, the creation of the State Children's Health Insurance Program (SCHIP) in 1997, the 2003 creation of a prescription drug benefit under Medicare, and the continuing saga of tens of millions of Americans who lack health insurance. While significant progress was made during the last decade of the twentieth century and the first decade of the twenty-first to help seniors meet their drug needs and assist children in securing basic services, the twin quandaries of some 45 million uninsured and continually rising costs still loom. It would seem that if these crippling problems are to be solved, an incremental approach will provide the way forward. For better or worse, attacking the problems one piece at a time may be our future.

REGULATING PRIVATE INSURANCE CAUTIOUSLY

As explained in Chapter 6, a chief criticism of the Clinton plan was its potential for limiting choice, in terms of both the available providers and the services they might be permitted to offer. The long-running argument about the sacred doctor-patient relationship had been made so often that a person might have been forgiven for not noticing that private insurance carriers had been limiting choice ever since the modern expansion of HMOs in the 1970s. As enrollment in HMOs grew rapidly during the mid-1990s and the medical rate of inflation continued apace, HMOs' incentive to limit patients' use of services intensified. Stories of services denied became commonplace, and an interesting irony came into view. What government was denied the opportunity to potentially do under publicly managed competition, private insurance carriers began to accomplish with disturbing regularity. New mothers and their children were hustled out of hospitals within 24 hours of delivery. Costly treatments were denied. Certain diagnostic tests were placed out of bounds for most patients. While these changes were associated with a brief period of stabilized medical inflation, they also created horror stories from patients who suffered tragic outcomes. Congress considered enacting a patient bill of rights but failed to deliver. Progress instead occurred in the states. Many state governments stepped in to fill the gap, passing patient bills of rights and various other regulations on insurance companies operating within their borders. During 1995 alone, some 250 protective bills were proposed in state legislatures. In 1996 that figure exceeded 1,000. By the end of the 1990s some 900 of these bills had become state laws. Targeting a popular point of objection, at least 30 states passed minimum hospital stay mandates and about as many required HMOs to report on the quality of care they delivered. Seventeen states established quality-of-care standards that HMOs were expected to meet. Twelve required external arbitration for disagreements between the enrollees and the HMO, and 18 established ombudsman offices to receive grievances. Many states prohibited nondoctors from making care decisions. By 1996, 18 states had prohibited so-called gag rules, provisions by which HMOs might prohibit doctors from discussing certain kinds of alternative treatments that may prove costly. Prohibitions on gag rules were probably unnecessary, as HMOs realized that such limitations were not only unfeasible (doctors were unlikely to cooperate) but also sufficiently controversial as to be political dynamite. By 1997, any earlier gag rules had disappeared from HMO contracts, according to a study by the U.S. General Accounting Office that year that examined the contracts of 529 HMOs and found no limits on the information doctors could share with patients. This wave of state legislation was far-reaching. By 2001 all but three states had enacted some type of protective legislation for patients.[1]

For its part, in 1997 Congress took the rather easy step of including a ban on gag provisions in HMO contracts, but it failed to enact anything more sweeping.[2] Instead, HMOs took proactive stances, regulating themselves by

becoming more transparent regarding compensation practices they main-
tained with their member providers and, most important, by adopting more
permissive stances toward the range of services they would cover. Complaints
declined in the late 1990s, but so did the modest cost savings—estimated at
5 to 10 percent—that had been achieved during the mid-1990s due to the
intervention of HMOs.[3]

Although the previous public furor over HMO behavior settled somewhat,
disagreements continued and litigation was still common. The tendency of
courts during this time to limit or deny patients' rights to sue their HMOs led
Congress to revisit the matter in 1999. That year the House narrowly passed a
patient bill of rights, but the measure failed in the Senate. Debate during 2000
did not lead to either chamber approving legislation in this area. Not to be dis-
suaded, proponents of a federal patients' bill of rights reintroduced a measure
in 2001, and they managed to get separate versions of the bill through both
House and Senate. However, the two chambers could not reach a compromise.[4]

The disagreements between Democrats, who generally favored more
extensive patient rights to sue, and Republicans, who tended to hold less permissive views, played out in terms of individual rights versus concerns over
rising insurance rates as a result of the cost of jury awards. Republican Senator
Don Nickles of Oklahoma argued in 2000 that a permissive bill would produce a "dramatic, draconian increase in the uninsured" by running up insurance costs, which would be passed on to employers.[5] Indeed, a 1999 survey of
employers had found that one-third of them said that they would likely drop
worker insurance if premium prices rose much more.[6]

As financially practical as the Republican position might have been at the
time, some within the party realized the political liability attached to that stance.
Republican campaign professional Scott Reed, who had managed Bob Dole's
1996 presidential campaign, suggested in an op-ed column in the *Augusta*
(GA) *Chronicle* in June 2000 that Republicans should handle this issue with
great care. He referred to public opinion polling that found that more than
80 percent of Americans supported a right to sue their HMOs for damages
resulting from denied coverage. Reed noted that "the Democrats' successful portrayal of Republicans as defenders of indefensible HMOs has hurt."[7] Painful or
not, the vast majority of Senate Republicans opposed the patient bill of rights
when it came to a vote that month. The Senate narrowly defeated the bill by a
vote of 51–48, with only four GOP members voting for it.

Aside from the heat and passion this issue generated on the part of consumers and politicians, another perspective argues that we might instead consider
the limits imposed by HMOs as rational. In 1999 a presidential commission
reported that medical procedures that lack a scientific basis may account for
30 percent of all medical spending in the United States, implying that many

of the services HMOs decline to cover are in fact nontherapeutic. In that report, Stanford University economist and member of Clinton's healthcare team, Alain Enthoven, noted that "the country risks making a terrible mistake if it overacts and treats every denial as an assault on patients. Denials are a necessary feature of a well-run plan."[8] Whether consumers want to move beyond their outrage when their HMO denies coverage for a procedure is, of course, not a matter for such cool analysis. Feeling the anger and hoping to reduce the number of suits they faced, Empire Blue Cross and Blue Shield, among other HMOs during the late 1990s, began to use outside expert panels to decide whether a particular procedure would be appropriate in a given circumstance.[9] Doctors also attempted to defuse the situation by not always being completely forthright with HMOs. A 1998 survey of doctors found that more than one-third of them had at least once deceived insurance companies in order to secure approval for treatments they believed were necessary.[10] For all their promise, HMOs faced severe challenges in delivering the savings and coherency their proponents had promised.

A second issue left lingering in the wake of the failure of the Clinton plan was the matter of insurance portability. Stories of workers trapped in underperforming jobs because of their fear of losing their employer-sponsored health insurance, and of otherwise eligible individuals being denied insurance coverage due to preexisting health conditions, meant that the rates of frictional unemployment and underemployment were higher than they should have been. The Clinton plan had proposed limits on the obstacles insurance companies could impose, but without those becoming law these discriminatory practices flourished.

A partial solution came in the form of a bill sponsored by Republican Senator Nancy Kassebaum and Democrat Edward Kennedy. Signed into law in August 1996, this act limited the ability of private insurers to deny sales of policies to workers in transition and those with preexisting conditions. Insurers could no longer deny group coverage beyond 12 months to a person who had developed a health condition within the six-month period before an application was made for the new coverage. The law also required insurers that sell individual policies to sell them to individuals so long as those persons meet three criteria: the person had prior coverage for at least 18 months, the person was not eligible for coverage under any group plan, and the person had exhausted their extended coverage from their previous employer. Insurers were prohibited from refusing coverage based on health considerations, and the law required insurers who sell in the small-group insurance market—ranging from 2 to 50 workers— to sell policies to all employers who request to purchase such a policy.[11]

The Kassebaum-Kennedy bill moved slowly through Congress, in large part because of the resistance of the insurance lobby. Insurers were concerned about required issuance of policies to individuals outside the employer-based group market. Because those people tend to be more expensive to insure, the industry resisted requirements to do so.[12] Attempting to address related objections, the House Republican version of the bill included caps on medical malpractice awards and prohibited certain kinds of state regulation of the insurance industry, two issues not addressed in the Senate bill. In cross-chamber negotiations, these two provisions were deleted. One other significant provision from the House Republican version was a tax incentive to create medical savings accounts, similar to individual retirement accounts but for medical expenses. A few years earlier, this idea had become a favorite of Republicans and advocates of consumer-driven healthcare financing, but it troubled Senator Kennedy because of his concerns about how wealthy and healthy people might opt out of the private insurance market, leaving behind those who needed more services and who would be costlier to underwrite. In response, the final bill limited medical savings accounts to 750,000 individuals who either worked at firms with fewer than 50 employees or who were self-employed.[13]

The idea of medical savings accounts was the brainchild of John Goodman, who had unsuccessfully tried to sell the idea to congressional Republicans back in 1990. In 1994 Senator Phil Gramm took an interest in Goodman's idea, just as congressional Republicans were searching for an alternative to the Clinton plan. Introducing Goodman to some of his Senate colleagues, Gramm called medical savings accounts "the only new healthcare idea [I have] seen in over 20 years."[14] As part of the Kassebaum-Kennedy bill, the idea of medical savings accounts helped sweeten a piece of regulatory legislation that was otherwise proving to be a difficult pill to swallow for many Republicans. Kennedy and others likewise found the savings accounts objectionable, but they were placated by this provision being enacted only as a four-year pilot program. Individuals would be permitted to place money in a tax-free account to be used for medical services in lieu of purchasing traditional insurance. As a precondition, individuals would be required to purchase a high deductible insurance policy. Funds could be rolled over from year to year, as opposed to the use-it-or-lose-it rule for flexible spending accounts. Small employers were encouraged to sponsor these plans, though relatively few of them did in the early years. A lack of familiarity may have been one reason, though another likely explanation is that owners and managers at small companies are the kind of people who often find themselves lacking the time to attend to such matters. As one observer noted, these employers are typically "not innovators . . . because they don't have time to think about it."[15] As of the end of 1997 only 41,000 accounts had been opened, far below the rather low ceiling of 750,000 set by the legislation.[16]

Despite this modest beginning, health savings accounts (HSAs) had caught the imagination of conservatives, who managed to incorporate an enlargement of the program in the 2003 legislation most famously known for creating a prescription drug benefit under Medicare (more on this later). Under this enhanced version, anyone is permitted to deposit up to $2,850 and families up to $5,650 annually into a health savings account. Funds may be invested in stocks, bonds, or other interest-bearing vehicles. Like the pilot program, this newer version of HSAs requires enrollees to purchase a high deductible insurance policy to cover catastrophic illness.

Health savings accounts grew in popularity. As of 2007 approximately 25 percent of employers sponsored HSAs, with many employers willing to contribute to these accounts. Contributions are tax exempt for both workers and employers, and for companies that chose to contribute, this allows them to reduce its health insurance liability. Some employers have dropped their traditional insurance completely in favor of HSAs. Wendy's International (the restaurateur) made this shift in 2005.[17] Despite the fact that HSAs make sense mainly for people who are healthy and who can tolerate the complexities of estimating future expenses, enrollment in them rose from 438,000 in late 2004 to 6.1 million at the beginning of 2008. An analysis of 2005 tax data from the Internal Revenue Service found that people using HSAs had significantly higher income than others. HSA users had an average adjusted gross income of $139,000, compared to $57,000 for those without. Further, 41 percent did not withdraw any money from their accounts that year.[18] Clearly, HSAs are not plans that appeal so strongly to those with modest incomes. They do, however, provide an attractive tax shelter for those who can afford to accumulate enough savings to effectively become self-insured (bearing in mind the continuation of the high-deductible, catastrophic policy requirement). Because funds may be withdrawn after age 65 for any purpose, HSAs provide a vehicle for long-term savings.[19]

Whether HSAs will provide a model for rethinking healthcare financing more broadly in a consumer-driven direction remains an open question. Certainly, the expansion of HSAs in recent years, when combined with some other developments, particularly the structure of the prescription drug benefit for Medicare beneficiaries, suggests that a consensus has established a firm hold on policy makers that blends public and private tools while clearly privileging the latter.

THE CONSUMER-DRIVEN MOVEMENT AS A CHALLENGE TO MEDICARE

The convergence of the consumer-driven healthcare movement with the sharp turn to the political Right taken by the Republican Party in the mid-1990s produced quite a lot of discussion about how to refashion Medicare, the federal government's single largest health program, into a tool for senior citizens—behaving as utility-maximizing consumers—to use more efficiently.

Part of the impetus behind this effort surely had to do with a desire to cut federal spending, pure and simple. However, another important philosophical consideration was also at work. Many conservatives in Congress wanted Medicare's beneficiaries to become more directly responsible for the way Medicare's funds would be used by making those dollars feel much more like part of a limited individual resource. While ultimately unsuccessful, the Republican call to transform Medicare was part of a larger ideological agenda that has gained considerable political traction and that is likely to condition future debates over healthcare reform. Treating citizens like consumers, despite its controversial nature in various respects, has become mainstream.

The 1995 challenge to Medicare's long-standing entitlement structure stands in fairly sharp contrast to its history. From its creation in 1965 through the early 1990s, political consensus governed the Medicare program. Healthcare analyst Jonathan Oberlander writes that this long-lasting consensus hinged on three points: first, both political parties broadly agreed on policy directions; second, political struggles over Medicare rarely triggered protracted public debates; and third, because both parties agreed on the program's fundamental principles, they went on to agree substantially on the larger vision, that Medicare should be a universal and federally funded entitlement. This is, at its core, a liberal consensus. However, when attacked in the mid-1990s, this consensus came unraveled not as a result of public opinion movement, but rather because of changes in the outlooks of political elites.[20] The period of open political conflict over Medicare passed, but the urge to treat patients more like shoppers has continued.

The fight over Medicare burst onto the national stage in the spring and summer of 1995 when Republicans proposed imposing individual spending limits and other significant cost-saving reforms. House Speaker Newt Gingrich's proposal was to reduce Medicare spending by approximately 30 percent, or $270 billion over the coming seven years, in an effort to prevent the program from becoming insolvent. An internal memo from the Ways and Means Committee obtained by journalists in August sketched plans to double the cost of premiums, raise annual deductibles, and possibly offer beneficiaries the option of receiving their Medicare benefits in the form of vouchers instead of the open-ended commitment the program has been since its inception.[21] Republicans insisted that these were merely options to consider but that significant steps would be needed to preserve the program into the future. Democrats accused them of attempting to destroy the entitlement basis of Medicare funding. Critics argued that these changes would draw off the healthy and wealthy participants in Medicare, turning it into more of a welfare program.[22]

For their part, Americans were wary of the idea of Medicare vouchers. When pollsters asked about converting Medicare to a voucher system, respondents voiced strong disapproval of the idea. A May 1995 survey found that 60 percent opposed vouchers compared to only 35 percent in favor.[23] Later in the summer when questions posed the possibility that recipients could keep any unspent portion of the voucher as cash, respondents were more evenly split, with 46 percent favoring the idea versus 43 percent opposed. Eleven percent remained unsure.[24]

Public skepticism aside, the House of Representatives approved a reduction in the rate of growth equaling $282 billion for Medicare and another $184 billion for Medicaid. The Senate followed, approving cuts of $256 billion for Medicare and $175 billion for Medicaid.[25] President Clinton's vetoes of those changes ultimately led to smaller reductions in the projected rate of growth and prompted House Republicans to focus their efforts on more incremental changes that could be made elsewhere. Medical savings accounts under the Kassebaum-Kennedy Act were part of this system, as was the creation of Medicare Part C or Medicare+Choice under the Balanced Budget Act of 1997. This allowed beneficiaries to choose between traditional Medicare, HMOs, and preferred-provider organizations.[26]

The intellectual justification for treating patients like shoppers has its modern genesis in studies sponsored by researchers working at such conservative or libertarian centers as the Heritage Foundation, the American Enterprise Institute, the Cato Institute, and the National Center for Policy Analysis.[27] A handful of academics, such as Regina Herzlinger of Harvard University, Mark Pauly of the University of Pennsylvania, and Richard Epstein of the University of Chicago, have also elaborated on the consumer-driven perspective in their writings. This is not a homogenous group. Epstein's strong libertarianism and consequent opposition to public welfare—such as Medicare and Medicaid—programs sets him apart from others in the larger consumer-driven movement. Others are content to tinker at the edges with incentives for more selective consumption.[28] Epstein's argument aside, a chief complaint from this group is that government programs are wasteful in part because they provide excessive insurance. The consumer-driven perspective extends the moral hazard argument to claim that many people engage in risky behaviors because they have too much health insurance. If instead, individuals had to pay out of pocket, they would smoke and drink less and would take better care of themselves.[29] In a nation where nearly 30 percent of people are obese—which brings on higher rates of heart disease, diabetes, osteoarthritis, liver disease, and pulmonary problems—this argument has some appeal. Given the temptation to live recklessly, in the eyes of advocates of a consumer-driven market, this concern tends to trump the more widely discussed problem of the tens of millions who lack health insurance. However, for them "the uninsured are not the problem; the overinsured are."[30]

In this framework, turning Medicare into a voucher program is seen as an incentive for senior citizens not only to shop for the cheapest insurance they can find, specifically, to not buy too much of it, but also to lead healthier lives. Of course, this perspective arguably underappreciates the need for basic medical services that exists apart from consumers' preferences for it. Purchasing basic health care, after all, is not like purchasing luxury goods.[31] As Timothy Jost has written, "a common troupe in the consumer-driven literature is to liken first-dollar health insurance coverage to first-dollar coverage for car maintenance, housing costs, or restaurant dining, which, they argue, would lead to wanton abuse. . . . This analogy ignores, of course, the fact that health care is usually time-consuming, inconvenient, unpleasant, uncomfortable, and sometimes just plain painful. A few people do pathologically pursue health care services, but most of us have better things to do. Designer prescription sunglasses, evoked by some advocates to epitomize health care consumption, are in fact not typical of health care products and services."[32] Recall that the criticisms of excessive consumption and associated health outcomes typically compare moderate levels of service use to very high levels of service use, not outcomes of those with regular access to services to those who lack it.[33]

One other perspective on the consumer-driven idea comes from a group of physicians interviewed in McAllen, Texas, in 2009 for what turned out to be a widely read article in the *New Yorker* magazine. The doctors were asked to imagine a negotiation over price between patients and their physicians. "A cardiologist tells an elderly woman that she needs bypass surgery and had Dr. Dyke see her. They discuss the blockages in her heart, the operation, the risks. And now they're supposed to haggle over the price as if he were selling a rug in a souk? 'I'll do three vessels for thirty thousand, but if you take four I'll throw in an extra night in the I.C.U.'—that sort of thing? Dyke shook his head. 'Who comes up with this stuff?' he asked. 'Any plan that relies on the sheep to negotiate with the wolves is doomed to failure.'"[34]

THE 1997 CREATION OF THE STATE CHILDREN'S HEALTH INSURANCE PROGRAM

Despite the growing support among some politicians and analysts for a more consumer-driven approach to health financing, the idea of insuring the vulnerable still carries considerable weight. This is particularly true regarding children. In this context and despite the essentially stable strength of conservative Republicans in Congress beyond the 1996 elections, calls for the government to do more for uninsured children proved successful. Congress passed, and states voluntarily adopted the SCHIP, which provides federal funds to states for the purpose of covering medical costs. SCHIP can be thought of as essentially an expansion of Medicaid. It targets low- to moderate-income children and is implemented by states using a combination of state and federal dollars to finance it.[35] At the program's outset, states were invited to cover children who did not have private health insurance and who lived in families that were not eligible for Medicaid but with income below 200 percent of the federal poverty rate. States could cover children in families with income above this level at their own expense.[36] As of spring 2009, the highest state income threshold was 300 percent of the federal poverty rate for children under age 1 in Maryland, Vermont, New Hampshire, and Hawaii.[37] States must fund a portion of the program expense, but in return they receive as much as or more than that amount of investment in federal money. In part due to the generosity of the funding arrangement, SCHIP spread quickly. All 50 states adopted it within its first two years.[38] At the time of its creation, SCHIP was expected to insure approximately five million of the nation's 10 million uninsured children at a cost of $20 billion over five years.[39] By 2004 enrollment reached just over six million.[40]

One of the concerns voiced early in this program's life was that parents would save themselves money by using SCHIP to replace their private insurance, a phenomenon referred to as crowding out. Evidence from a variety of studies seems to indicate that very little crowding out occurs, as the vast majority of enrolled children did not in fact previously have private insurance. Only about one-third of children on SCHIP have a parent who enjoys health insurance at work, so at maximum crowding out can only occur in about one-third of all cases. The likely rate is lower than this because many parents at this income level work for employers who do not offer insurance for employees' dependents.[41] However, to address this issue nearly all states adopted waiting periods for children who previously had private insurance in order to minimize this behavior.

SCHIP proved popular with states and with low- to moderate-income parents. Between 1997 and 2003, enrollment grew quickly before leveling off. The take-up rate for SCHIP and Medicaid combined, that is, the portion of eligible children who are actually enrolled, reached approximately 70 percent by 2003. Encouragingly, it grew most rapidly in areas where the rates of insurance among children were previously low.[42]

SCHIP was due for reauthorization in 2007 (for the 2008 fiscal year). Congressional Democrats sought to expand it to provide funding to states that wanted to raise their income thresholds above the then-current 200 percent level. Given that the Congressional Budget Office estimated that the program in its present configuration would have required some 12 billion additional dollars merely to continue the current level of coverage from 2008 through 2012, this began to seem like an expensive proposition.[43] However, Democrats stressed that several million children remained without insurance and that a program expansion could whittle away at that problem. President Bush countered that this push was an effort to make SCHIP into something it was never intended to be and that it was not supposed to cover effectively middle-class children.

The public was squarely behind the Democrats in wanting to expand SCHIP. Typical of many polls on this issue, one in early October 2007 found that 67 percent of respondents thought that the government was spending too little on health insurance for children. Further, when asked directly about support for expanding SCHIP, 70 percent of respondents supported it, compared to only 26 percent who opposed.[44]

These findings, perhaps not surprisingly, did not change the president's mind. He and his allies pointed out that by proposing that federal funding be available to families at 300 percent of the poverty level, Democrats were willing to extend help to children whose parents earn just over $61,000 each year, an expansion that called for some $50 billion in additional spending over the coming five years. He was willing to support a more modest expansion, but not as large as that advocated by congressional Democrats. Sticking to his position, Bush twice vetoed the expansion, once in October and again in December 2007. The president called the Democrats' effort "misguided" and said that it "would have expanded SCHIP to higher-income households while increasing taxes."[45] The taxes he was referring to were mainly cigarette taxes, something many congressional Republicans objected to as well. Seeing no possibility of overcoming the president's veto, the reauthorization bill was revised to trim Medicare spending to pay for a more modest SCHIP expansion.[46] This new version extended SCHIP through March 2009. The president signed it into law on December 29, 2007.

Later, with a Democrat in the White House, Congress sent President Obama legislation in February 2009 to expand SCHIP from its present level of some seven million children to 11 million. Health groups cheered the move. American Hospital Association President Richard Umbdenstock said that "Congress and the administration rightly recognize that, like education, healthcare is a basic prerequisite for kids to have a productive future. America's hospitals strongly support the reauthorization of SCHIP."[47] This was an easy bill for medical providers to support. Even if states' reimbursement rates under SCHIP are lower than they would like, doctors and hospitals clearly see the benefit of ensuring better basic care and preventative services with some payment rather than no payment. With this expansion in place, one more piece of a very complicated puzzle had fallen into place.

THE CREATION OF A MEDICARE PRESCRIPTION DRUG BENEFIT

Democrats had long hoped to add an outpatient prescription drug component to Medicare, but the expense had proven an obstacle for members of

Congress and presidents, and the prospect of accompanying price controls (which did not occur in 2003) had dampened support for the idea in the pharmaceutical industry.[48] The short-lived catastrophic coverage part of the program in the late 1980s had included this benefit, but that ended along with the controversial higher premium that was part of the package. In 2003 the Bush White House saw in a prescription drug benefit an opportunity to score points with seniors at a time when the president's approval rating among them was declining. Most congressional Republicans viewed a drug benefit as a powerful issue to carry them through the 2004 elections. Some Democrats and their natural allies, including the AARP, found themselves unhappy with some of the Republican ideas for Medicare but uncomfortable in obstructing this long-sought benefit. Some fiscal conservatives complained about the extent of government involvement and spending in this package, but they were essentially voices in the political wilderness this time around. In the end, the addition of a drug benefit for Medicare was an uneasy marriage between a trusted though imperfect program and some newer ideas that have brought some tremendous benefits to many but potentially at a price that will prove severely challenging in the near term.

Upon final passage, the Medicare Prescription Drug, Improvement, and Modernization Act of 2003 saw a deep partisan divide, with the vast majority of Democrats opposing it and nearly all Republicans in support. Though complicated, the crux of the disagreement was about Republican ideas to move Medicare toward a managed care program built on government-subsidized premiums paid to private insurers and the design of the drug benefit itself. Regarding managed care, the initial House version of the bill had as its goal to move Medicare to a premium support model—one in which beneficiaries would receive a government subsidy to purchase private insurance. This was premised on the idea that private insurers could cover seniors more efficiently than does government, for the same reasons so many employers turned to managed care in the 1990s. Many seniors, however, objected to what they believed was a move to privatize Medicare.[49] South Dakota Senator Tom Daschle complained at the end of July 2003 that a move to a premium support model is "alien to our concept of Medicare" and that he fervently hoped that the more moderate Senate version of the bill would prevail in the end.[50]

Regarding the drug benefit, early in negotiations both chambers settled on a three-tier structure. Beneficiaries would pay one-quarter of their drug costs up to some level. They would then become responsible for all of their costs up to some higher level. Beyond this, fairly high threshold government assistance would resume, covering nearly all additional costs. Precise thresholds were refined throughout the summer and fall. In the end, recipients would be responsible for 25 percent up to $2,250 each year. Expenses between that level and $5,100 would fall entirely on recipients (the so-called doughnut hole in coverage). Beyond $5,100 in drug expenses each year, Medicare would pay 95 percent. Many Democrats complained that the doughnut hole would leave vulnerable seniors without help just at the point when their annual drug bills became genuinely burdensome. However, Republican architects of the House and Senate bills shied away from attempting comprehensive coverage due to its high projected costs.

To inject some market flavor into this program, an annual deductible of $250 would apply to all but the lowest income beneficiaries, and seniors would be required to select a formulary that best fit their needs, with most drug plans costing between $30 and $70 per month. Helping the elderly to select an appropriate plan required considerable public education efforts by the Department of Health and Human Services. Most important, and this was probably the most controversial part of the package, the final version of the bill also included a pilot program that would operate in up to six metropolitan areas, to be selected by the secretary of Health and Human Services, in which seniors could enroll in managed care plans that would directly compete with Medicare. This was the toned-down version of what House Republicans had written into their version of the bill.[51] Many if not most Democrats saw in this provision a thinly veiled attempt to privatize Medicare, a move that potentially threatened to deprive seniors of the assurance of coverage the program had always provided.

In contrast to these pro-market provisions, and much to the dismay of many observers, the final bill prohibited the Department of Health and Human Services from negotiating drug prices, like the Veteran's Administration and the Department of Defense do for their clients, and did not allow for drug reimportation from other nations.[52] The federal government would not be permitted to use its massive purchasing power to drive down prices. Blame for these anticompetitive provisions were laid at the doorstep of millions of dollars of campaign contributions from pharmaceutical companies to Republicans over the years. Acknowledging the coup that these protections represented, a drug industry lobbyist said of the legislation that "this is a huge victory."[53] Congress and the Food and Drug Administration had wrestled with the reimportation issue for years, and while seniors will continue seeking drugs internationally, especially from Canada, the 2003 legislation ensured that the vast majority of the increased demand for prescription medications would fall to U.S. markets.

During the negotiations, the leadership of the AARP found itself in a difficult position, wanting to support the addition of a prescription drug benefit but also desirous of preserving traditional Medicare. Many observers wondered out loud during the summer of 2003 if the AARP had forgotten the drubbing it suffered at its members' hands in the late 1980s when disgruntled seniors took out their frustrations on the advocacy organization over its support for the catastrophic care program that imposed increased premiums for some higher-income beneficiaries. Entering the game rather late this time around, the AARP's November endorsement of the bill seemed to lack discernment of the particulars of the pending legislation. Its ads said, "Congress, you made a good start [by getting bills through both chambers]. Now finish the job. We ask that you keep your promise and add prescription drug coverage to Medicare."[54] To this, a Democratic staffer in Congress criticized the lack of incisiveness, saying, "I don't at all understand what the use is in spending tons of money" to encourage Congress to pass a bill. "It matters what's in it."[55] By not weighing in on the specifics the group ran the risk of another debacle like that of 1988. Within a day of its endorsement, the AARP's online message board was flooded with negative feedback from members. They were angry over what they saw as the organization's failure to discern seniors' interests. One left a note reading, "not only did you do a great disservice to your members, you're now spending $7 million [on advertising] to try to justify it. Shame on you!"[56] Following this episode, some 60,000 AARP members either dropped their membership or elected not to renew it.[57]

Despite misgivings on various fronts, Congress passed the final bill by narrow margins (220–215 in the House and 54–44 in the Senate) during the last week of November, and the president signed it into law on December 8, 2003.[58] Within two months news emerged that the cost estimate provided by the administration was faulty. At the time of passage members of Congress worked with a price tag of $395 billion over 10 years, a figure that was conveniently 5 billion below a Senate budget resolution that, if violated, would likely have triggered a procedural challenge to the bill. However, Richard Foster, the chief actuary at the Department of Health and Human Services, had realized in the summer of 2003 that a better estimate would be closer to $535 billion. His information was suppressed by Thomas Scully, the administrator of the Centers for Medicare and Medicaid Services, who threatened Foster with being terminated if he released the revised figure.[59] A later investigation determined that Scully had perhaps acted improperly but that he broke no laws. Members of Congress minimally protested the intentionally incorrect information from the administration, but it was too late to do much about it. In February 2005 the administration provided yet another revised estimate, this one of $720 billion.[60] As if this cost escalation were not enough, because of a delay in implementation from the time of passage in late 2003 until 2006 when the full range of benefits would actually begin, the 10-year budget includes only eight years of the program, artificially depressing the cost estimate. Critics howled over the gaming of the budget figures, and conservative Heritage Foundation's director of health policy issues complained that "there's no excuse for what the administration did."[61] Support for the law among the senior citizens at the time of its signing remained weak, with nearly half (47%) of them voicing opposition and only 26 percent in favor. Support among the public as a whole was similarly low.[62]

The many winners under this legislation included the Bush administration, at least in the short term, hospitals, who saw an increase in Medicare payments under other provisions of the law, seniors, especially those whose drug costs fall mainly within covered expense ranges, and certainly the pharmaceutical industry, which has seen an uptick in demand and payment for its products. Losers arguably include the taxpayers who will fund this tremendously expensive program that has few cost controls built in. Senator Tom Daschle was not alone in labeling this as "basically a corporate welfare bill for drug companies and HMOs."[63] Given rising drug prices, an aging population, and the increasing use of drug therapies, the estimates generated in 2003 and 2004 may, even in the short run, bear little resemblance to the program's true cost.

THE SUM OF THE PARTS

The enactment of drug coverage for seniors, consumer protections for those attempting to maintain or purchase private insurance, and government health insurance for children in low- to moderate-income families has certainly benefited millions of Americans over the past decade. Political actors across the ideological spectrum tend to believe that these have been useful steps in bridging the gaps that stand between the nation's most vulnerable populations and the basic and preventative care they need and that consumers face a more fair fight when they rely on the private insurance market in times of sickness or injury.

The nagging problems of coverage and cost, however, still persist and show no signs of reversing. Depending on how one counts, between 45 and 55 million Americans lack health insurance, either on a year-round basis (the lower figure) or for at least part of the year (the higher figure). In round terms, this accounts for some 17 percent of the population. The opportunities for inefficient cost-shifting, missed preventative care, expensive visits to emergency rooms instead of more routine visits to doctors' offices, and quality care that could improve and lengthen lives are vast, given the size of the uninsured population.[64]

The composition of this pool has changed somewhat over the years. In the 1960s a solid majority of the uninsured were poor. That is still true today (some 70% of the uninsured are poor), but increasingly the ranks of the uninsured are middle-class people and those who work at least part time.

Nearly three-quarters of uninsured adults are employed. Most of the nonaged uninsured work full-time but for employers who cannot or chose not to provide insurance. As more Americans work for smaller firms, they encounter insurance as an employment benefit less frequently. Nearly all companies with more than 1,000 workers provide insurance (98.6% of them in 2003), but only two-thirds of those with between 10 and 24 workers do. A little more than one-third of firms with fewer than 10 employees offer insurance. The fixed costs of administration and marketing and the risk of adverse selection (i.e., picking up chronically sick workers whose load is shared among fewer coworkers) provide disincentives to smaller employers.[65] The shift away from manufacturing has advanced this trend, as has the decline in the number of unionized workplaces. For workers, recent changes have been dramatic. In 2000, 67 percent of Americans with insurance obtained it through their employer or from the employer of a household member. By 2004 that figure had fallen to 63 percent. One of the distressing results is that approximately one out of five of the uninsured is a child.[66]

Arguing for universal coverage does not tend to elicit the objections that it used to. Even Republican strategists tend to respond with questions about how to achieve universalism rather than the wisdom of the goal itself. This gradual shift toward thinking of healthcare provision as a basic right of citizenship has been reflected not only in government actions, as described here, but also in public opinion. When compared to spending in other areas, Americans tend to rank health more highly. Also, its ranking has risen in recent years. Figure 7.1 shows the percentage of respondents to the General Social Survey who believe that we spend too little on health care, Social Security, assistance to the poor, the environment, and education from 1991 to 2008. (Response options included that we are spending "too little," "about the right amount," or "too much.") The only close competitor is education, which received strong support for additional spending from the public throughout the 1990s, though health care has surpassed it in most of the recent years of the survey. Even preferences for spending on Social Security, which have increased sharply since 1993, still remain some 10 percentage points below Americans' preferences for increased spending on health care.

Given this level of popular support for health spending, it is understandable that Congress has taken significant strides to fill some of the gaps in insurance coverage that have endured over the years. Proponents of this incremental approach can claim some victories. However, the large and slowly growing uninsured population, together with the rising percentage of national wealth that healthcare services consume, provides stubborn evidence that much work remains. The patchwork set of public and private programs that help Americans get the services they need work more or less well for most individuals within

Figure 7.1
Americans' Preferences for Spending on Health Care and Other Priorities

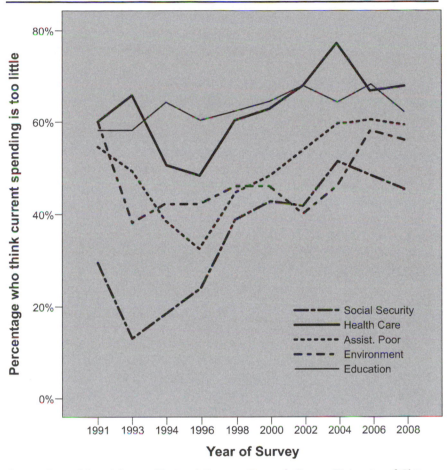

Source: General Social Survey, National Opinion Research Center, University of Chicago (1972–2008 cumulative data file). See endnote for question wording.[67]

targeted groups—children in low-income families, the elderly, and those who work for employers who sponsor insurance plans—but not for others. Their fragmentary nature leaves so many gaps that moving from childhood to adulthood, from one job to another, or from the workplace into retirement presents the risk of loss of benefits. This patchwork should probably not be considered a system, but rather a diverse assortment of programs that most Americans successfully navigate only with quite a bit of effort and a measure of luck. Moving toward a coherent system will require rethinking the answers to some of the questions discussed here, and that will be an exquisitely difficult political exercise. But it will also begin to address the needs of the one out of every six Americans who lives day to day in the fervent hope of not becoming sick.

NOTES

1. Schlesinger 2005, p. 114; Quadagno 2004, p. 830; Coombs 2005, p. 257; Budrys 2005, p. 129.
2. *Congressional Quarterly Almanac 1997*, pp. 6–12.
3. Funigiello 2005, p. 278.
4. Quadagno 2004, p. 830.
5. All quotes from Associated Press, "Senate GOP Votes Down Health Care Bill that Includes Broad Right to Sue HMOs," June 9, 2000.
6. Coombs 2005, pp. 242–243.
7. Scott Reed, "Patients' Rights Support a Wake-up Call for GOP," *Augusta Chronicle*, June 9, 2000, p. A-5.
8. Michael Weinstein, "Managed Care's Other Problem: It's Not What You Think," *New York Times*, February 28, 1999, sect. 4, p. 1.
9. Ibid.
10. Coombs 2005, p. 256.
11. *Congressional Quarterly Almanac 1996*, pp. 6–28.
12. Ibid.
13. Ibid, pp. 6–29; Amy Goldstein, "Republican Leaders Reach Deal on Medicare," *Washington Post*, November 16, 2003, p. A-1.
14. Matthew DoBias, "HAS Architect Sees More Opportunities," *Modern Healthcare*, June 19, 2006, p. 7.
15. Jennifer Steinhauer, "Curing What Ails Medical Savings Plan," *Plain Dealer* (Cleveland), September 11, 2000, p. 1-E.
16. U.S. General Accounting Office, "Medical Savings Accounts: Results from Surveys of Insurers," report # GAO/HEHS-99/34, December 1998.
17. Susan Straight, "Of Sickness and of Wealth," *Washington Post*, June 10, 2007, p. F-1.
18. U.S. General Accounting Office, "Health Savings Accounts," report # GA-08-802T, May 2008.
19. Jost 2007, p. 22.
20. Oberlander 2003, pp. 5–7.
21. Spencer Rich, "Medicare Premiums Would Soar under New Option in GOP Plan," *Washington Post*, August 12, 1995, p. A-8.
22. Oberlander 2003, p. 3; Funigiello 2005, p. 285.
23. "Which of these two descriptions comes closer to your view of what Medicare should look like in the year 2000? The Medicare program would remain as it is today, with a fixed set of benefits and the government providing individuals with a single insurance care. Medicare as know it would no longer exist, but rather people would receive from the government a check or voucher for a fixed amount each year and buy their own private health insurance policy." Sixty percent keep as is; 35 percent change to

voucher; 5 percent not sure. Poll by Harris and Associates, May 31 to June 5, 1995, $N = 1,383$.

24. "Another proposal is to replace Medicare with a system in which recipients would receive vouchers to purchase health insurance of their choice. If their choice costs more than the value of the voucher, the recipient would pay the difference. If it costs less, they would keep the difference. Do you favor or oppose this voucher system?" Forty-six percent favor, 43 percent oppose, 11 percent not sure. Poll by Yankelovich Partners, September 13 to 14, 1995, $N = 1,000$.

25. Smith 2002, pp. 80–82.

26. Oliver et al. 2004, p. 303.

27. Jost 2007, p. 27.

28. Ibid., p. 30; see Herzlinger 2004 for a collection of essays on the consumer-driven movement.

29. Jost 2007, p. 34, but importantly see also Herzlinger 1997, pp. 64–69, and Goodman and Musgrave 1992, p. 94.

30. Jost 2007, p. 35.

31. Ibid., p. 33.

32. Ibid., p. 35.

33. See Epstein 1997, pp. 156–157, for an example of this type of comparison without mention of the justification for the consequences of basic service provision.

34. Gawande 2009, p. 44.

35. Public Law # 105-33, the Balanced Budget Act of 1997.

36. See Herz et al. 2008 for a brief overview.

37. Kaiser Family Foundation interactive map available online at: www.state healthfacts.org (accessed June 27, 2009).

38. Swartz 2006, p. 35; Kenny and Yee 2007, pp. 356–357.

39. *Congressional Quarterly Almanac 1997*, pp. 6–12.

40. Herz et al. 2008.

41. Kenny and Yee 2007, p. 359.

42. Cunningham 2003; Kenny and Yee 2007, pp. 357–358.

43. Kenny and Yee 2007, p. 361.

44. "Congress is proposing to spend an additional $35 billion over the next five years in order to maintain coverage for those already in the program and to expand coverage to an additional 3.8 million uninsured children. The expansion would be financed by an increase in cigarette taxes. In general, would you say you support or oppose the increased funding for this program?" Seventy percent support, 26 percent oppose, 3 percent don't know ($N = 1527$, October 8–13, 2007).

45. *Congressional Quarterly Almanac 2007*, p. 12-8.

46. Ibid., p. 12-3.

47. Jennifer Lubell, "Boost for SCHIP," *Modern Healthcare*, February 9, 2009, p. 10.

48. Oliver et al. 2004, pp. 292–297.

49. Marilyn Werber Serafini, "A Prescription for Defeat," *National Journal*, August 30, 2003, pp. 2608–2617.

50. Richard Cohen, "For the Democrats, a Looming Dilemma," *National Journal*, August 30, 2003, p. 2621.

51. *Congressional Quarterly Almanac 2003*, pp. 11-3–11-13.

52. Relman 2007, pp. 84–85.

53. Marilyn Werber Serafini, "No Cure-All," *National Journal*, November 22, 2003, p. 3589.

54. Marilyn Werber Serafini, "A Senior Moment for AARP?" *National Journal*, September 20, 2003, p. 2883.

55. Ibid.

56. Serafini, "No Cure-All," p. 3587.

57. Oliver et al. 2004, p. 319.

58. *Congressional Quarterly Almanac 2003*, pp. 11–3. Public Law 108–173.

59. Oliver et al. 2004, pp. 315, 323.

60. Budrys 2005, p. 106.

61. Funigiello 2005, pp. 296–298 (quote on p. 296).

62. Oliver et al. 2004, pp. 283–354.

63. Serafini, "No Cure-All," p. 3587.

64. See Kaiser Family Foundation 2007 for a discussion of the causes and consequences of a large uninsured population.

65. Swartz 2006, pp. 52–55.

66. Ibid., chapter 1; Funigiello 2005, pp. 281–282.

67. "We are faced with many problems in this country, none of which can be solved easily or inexpensively. I'm going to name some of these problems, and for each one I'd like you to tell me whether you think we're spending too much money on it, too little money, or about the right amount. Are we spending too much, too little, or about the right amount on . . . health care."

8

Struggling toward a Healthcare System

How could Americans ignore the health needs of so many countrymen and still live with themselves? How could a society that prides itself on decency tolerate this degree of unfairness?

—David Rothman[1]

America did not pass comprehensive national health care reform in 1994 for the same reason it could not pass it in 1948, 1965, 1974, and 1978. The United States is the only democratic country that does not have a comprehensive national health insurance system because American political institutions are structurally biased against this kind of comprehensive reform.

—Sven Seinmo and Jon Watts[2]

As this book goes to press, Congress and the president have once again taken up the task of crafting legislation that strives toward universal healthcare coverage. In this political season, the fact that most Americans support the idea of universal coverage may either turn out to be one of the most important principles that motivates policy makers, or it may turn out to be largely irrelevant.

An enduring paradox in the debate over health politics is that while most Americans support universal care, we have not reached that goal because of our deep conflicts about how to achieve it, and our political institutions offer numerous venues for that conflict to thwart the smooth transmission of majority public opinion into policy. Traditionally these factors have been placed into two categories: attitudinal or cultural explanations in the first and institutional explanations in the second. Each bears a bit of revisiting.

To the great extent that many or even most Americans harbor ideas of rugged individualism and the existence of a clear track between self-application and personal achievement, the notion of government provision of access to medical services for all runs afoul of some deep-seated predispositions. Certainly, Americans widely adhere to a sense of humanitarianism, and this makes calls for some types of universal provision of basic services resonate politically.[3] But health services, even basic ones it would appear, have not quite achieved the status of a citizenship right, akin to public education or the protections enshrined in the Bill of Rights. Weak trust in government, periodically aggravated by scandals and inter- or intraparty conflict, further undermines confidence in and any inclination to look to the public sector as a source of provision, particularly given the tremendously complex nature of health care. This is precisely what gives antigovernment rhetoric its force. Recall the clever line from the 1993 essay in the *National Review* written by Dick Armey and Newt Gingrich: "If you like the way the Federal Government runs public housing and the state government runs the Department of Motor Vehicles, you'll love health care under the Clinton Plan."[4] By tapping into two hated examples of seemingly dysfunctional government bureaucracy and linking them to a proposal for government-organized health financing, opponents were able to tie a rather heavy weight around the neck of a meticulously designed, if arguably flawed, program to achieve universal coverage. Rather than seeing the Clinton plan, or any of the many proposals that went before it, as starting points for negotiations and refinement, antigovernment rhetoric helped doom those plans, leaving Americans to struggle with an increasingly bad status quo. Our poorly developed sense of social citizenship—that citizenship alone should denote rights to a certain level of social provision, just as it generally denotes the right to an education or a vote—certainly does nothing to mitigate a lack of confidence in government as a vehicle to take us to where most of us more or less agree we want to go: basic health services available to all.

Our fragmented political system also matters a great deal. Bicameralism, the Senate's frequently invoked supermajority requirement, interbranch conflicts, congressional committee jurisdictions and their resulting turf battles, and legislators who are pulled not only by constituents but also by powerful and well-endowed interest groups all combine to make passage of controversial, complex, and far-reaching legislation, if not impossible, at least exceedingly difficult. Consider the snail's pace of women's suffrage, civil rights legislation, and meaningful campaign finance reform. One perspective on this problem is that "American institutions were designed to be incompetent."[5] This is to argue that our political system was designed to work against revolution or even swift moving change through its incorporation of multiple veto points. The price we pay for this buffer against radicalism is the difficulty we have in addressing complex problems with bold solutions. A softer version of this view is that our system is one that moves decisively only when confronted with persistent supermajorities and that the rest of America's political evolution is characterized by incrementalism. In either formulation, our institutions often do us no favors when the time comes to move expeditiously in pursuit of pressing needs, especially when multiple streams of thought demand a place at the table. In years past the primary source of objections came from organized medicine, principally the AMA. Today, however, the main obstacle to progressive reform is the insurance industry, fearful of losing its lucrative position as part of a sector that accounts for approximately one-seventh of the nation's economy. Regardless of the source of objections, our political institutions provide plenty of venues to amplify those points of resistance.

The attitudinal and institutional explanations for the failure of comprehensive reform are only separate in a conceptual sense. As important as that separation may be, in practice the two explanations go hand in hand. Institutional obstacles matter so much precisely because of the attitudinal disagreements that fundamentally plague our healthcare discourse. Of course, the American founders did not design a fragmented political system in order to frustrate healthcare reform, but the effect has certainly been to create nearly insuperable obstacles for reform proponents. Lacking an overwhelmingly large public majority in support of any single approach, the attitudinal differences are magnified and perpetuated by our institutionally fragmented way of making law. In this sense, majority support for universalism may be beside the point when it comes to attempts to enact far-reaching reform.

However, that popular majority support still bears careful consideration. When asked in the spring of 2009 how high a priority it is for Congress and the president to guarantee universal coverage, 58 percent of respondents called it either the most important priority or one of the top two or three priorities facing the nation. Another 23 percent called it an important but not a top priority.[6] In a July 2009 poll 39 percent said that reforming health care should be "one of [Congress's and President Obama's] top priorities, and another 35 percent called it a "very important but not top priority."[7] This level of support explains the perennial interest in the issue. Of course, achieving health coverage for all would go a long way toward addressing the problems of cost shifting and of untreated illness and chronic conditions as obstacles to meaningful employment, and it would have salutary effects on children, as they would enjoy greater levels of preventative care. Universal access to medical care is a powerful idea indeed, but so too are efforts to target assistance to particular groups.

Targeting benefits at particularly needy or deserving groups has met with considerable success. On these many occasions large majorities have been able to agree, and once in place those programs have tended to foster strong constituencies that will fight for the preservation of those benefits. Medicare was created as a benefit to retired workers and for a vulnerable group with higher-than-average medical bills. Senior citizens have effectively rallied behind it on various occasions. Although it targets the poor, medical providers and state governments come to the defense of Medicaid when deep cuts are threatened. Similarly, Americans strongly supported the expansion of SCHIP as a way of helping children, even if those children did not all come from desperately needy families. Targeting sharpens the argument for benefits, most effectively when the group in question is part of a narrative of deservingness or pity. Beginning in 1798, the federal government targeted assistance to disabled seamen. Workers who built the Panama Canal and the dams of the Tennessee Valley Authority enjoyed federal health coverage. Beginning in 1935 the federal Resettlement Administration, later called the Farm Security Administration, reimbursed doctors and dentists for services rendered to poor farmers. At its peak this program helped pay for services to some 600,000 people living in over 1,000 counties across the country.[8] Military veterans have long received pensions and medical care on an open-ended, if still imperfect, basis (consider the criticisms of the staff at Walter Reed Hospital during the Iraq War). Even Native Americans living on reservations received assistance from the 1910s forward.[9] Targeted benefits draw political strength from the rightness of helping the particular group in question. They do not rely on broader arguments about social citizenship or an obligation to help the undifferentiated other. In this respect, these programs are resilient, but collectively they are also fragmented and quite incomplete. This, however, is the American pattern.

While this pattern is perhaps understandable, government coverage of only select groups leaves large swaths of the population without access to care, and this approach thwarts efforts to achieve greater economies of scale. Two related problems flow from these shortcomings. First, a lack of regular access leads to poorer health and shorter lives. Second, inefficiencies in financing systems combined with generally rising costs threaten not only household but also government budgets, and they greatly stress private employers struggling to provide for their workers.

When uninsured people do obtain services, those services are often delayed. As a result, the conditions are often more expensive to treat. Hospitalizations result from conditions that could have been treated earlier in a doctor's office. A study of the uninsured in 2006 found that approximately one-quarter of them had recently foregone care, as contrasted with about

5 percent of insured adults. About one-quarter of the uninsured had put off filling a prescription. Missing care puts children in particular at risk for more serious illnesses later. Thirty-seven percent of uninsured children had gone two years or more since their last dental visit, compared to 13 percent of those with private insurance. Adults with insurance are at least 50 percent more likely than uninsured ones to receive timely preventative care. Uninsured adults who are admitted to hospitals are significantly more likely than insured ones to die there. A Kaiser Family Foundation study estimated that insuring those who are currently uninsured could reduce this group's mortality rate by between 10 and 25 percent. That translates to at least an additional 18,000 deaths in 2000 that otherwise would not have occurred.[10] An argument that one's use of medical services is really nothing more than a reflection of personal tastes would seem to miss the point of these figures. A basic level of service access is not simply one of convenience or taste. It translates to a matter of life and death for thousands of Americans every year.

If these figures are insufficient to animate reform conversations, distress over rising costs provides another reason to engage the issue. An undeniable reality is that expenditures on medical services have stressed the national economy and will continue to do so even more severely if the growth in this sector is not limited. Americans spent approximately $2.2 trillion on health in 2008. It is estimated that by 2014 that figure will reach $3.6 trillion.[11] Stated differently, Americans spent just over 16 percent of the gross domestic product on health in 2008, a figure that is projected to reach one-third by 2030. Not only does this create havoc for federal and state budgets, it also impacts employers to the extent that noticeably fewer of them now provide insurance for their workers. In 2000, 69 percent of employers offered it, but by 2005 that figure had dropped to 60 percent.[12] Among small businesses, that figure was closer to 55 percent in 2009, according to the National Federation of Independent Businesses.[13] Nearly everyone agrees that this is a completely unhealthy situation not only for small business owners but also for the country as a whole.

Critical as they are, these problems have not been sufficient to prompt members of Congress to set aside ideological axes, concerns over narrow issues, or short-term electoral strategies in favor of longer-term and more consequential solutions. Despite the upwardly spiraling healthcare costs that essentially constitute a slow-motion train wreck in progress, shared sacrifice has recently proven to be a hard sell, given the powerfully organized interests standing in opposition to reform. The very heated debates during 2009 and 2010 over government's role in the healthcare market highlighted some enduring concerns that make this one of the most intractable policy areas in American politics. Fears of a slippery slide into socialized medicine, incessantly

stoked by complaints of an imminent government takeover of health care, con-
flate the very real difference between government-funded health care and
government-provided health care. Under the main bills considered by the
U.S. House and Senate in 2009 and 2010, no medical providers would be com-
pelled to treat any patient. This fact, however, did little to assuage the panic and
hysteria surrounding what might have otherwise been a constructive public
conversation about reform. If it is true as a law of American politics that less-
complicated rhetoric forces out more-complicated rhetoric, the failure of
thoughtful bipartisanship on this issue at this time provided a dramatic illustra-
tion of this point.

Although the Democratically controlled Senate Finance Committee took
the lead in crafting a reform bill in early 2009, throughout most of the spring
and summer Republican members, by and large, stayed away from the negotiations. Democratic Senator Max Baucus's efforts to write a moderate bill
went unrewarded by the vast majority of his Republican colleagues, whose
opposition followed tactical advice offered by Republican public opinion
pollster Frank Luntz in a memo he distributed to GOP members in the
spring.[14] Luntz offered a softer version of William Kristol's 1993 strategy
memo, which had argued that allowing Democrats a legislative victory of this
magnitude would cement the partisan loyalties of working-class people for a
generation.[15] This time around the advice was for members of Congress to
acknowledge the problems many Americans face with their health care but
to shift the focus to the personal risks that he said would accompany a "Washington takeover" of health care managed by faceless bureaucrats, language
that was used repeatedly by reform opponents throughout the remainder of
2009, particularly in the town hall meetings held during Congress's August
recess.[16] By encouraging politicians and opinion leaders to focus on individuals' situations instead of on problems with the nation's healthcare system,
Luntz attempted to shift attention away from the inefficiencies of payment
systems, the tens of millions of uninsured, and the aggregate impact of
mounting medical expenditures. Luntz stated as his first point, "Abandon
and exile **ALL** references to the '*healthcare system*.'"[17] Framing the debate this
way likely leads people to be disinclined to consider broad public needs over
their own conditions. Because most insured Americans report being happy
with their medical providers and their health insurance plans, these insured
people will be less likely to take into account broad public needs in favor of
considering their own situations as individuals. In an effort to counter this,
President Obama's speech throughout this period frequently contained references to how those who are satisfied with their health insurance will be able to
keep it. The rhetorical battle was met.

The late summer's uproar from administration critics, including false claims that the pending legislation would compel senior citizens to discuss their own death plans with their doctors, marked a turning point in the larger debate. Elizabeth McCaughey, the Republican critic of the Clinton plan in the 1990s who by spring 2009 once again had healthcare reform in her sights, told talk show host and former presidential candidate Fred Thompson that "the Congress would make it mandatory—absolutely require—that every five years people in Medicare have a required counseling session that will tell them how to end their lives sooner."[18] No such requirement existed. Rather, the proposal was for Medicare to pay for discussion sessions between doctors and patients when the patients desire to talk about end-of-life issues. These sorts of discussions that routinely occur but which represent uncompensated care under Medicare would now be covered by the program. McCaughey's mendacity notwithstanding, the death panel discussion took on a life of its own through the late summer, likely representing to many conservative skeptics just how invasive reform legislation might be. This provision, as non-threatening as it was in reality, was dropped from the developing legislation, and by mid-August the administration began backing away from another highly controversial position, a government-run insurance option.[19] Other concessions would follow.

By this time, three House committees and two in the Senate had made significant progress in developing bills. While the details varied, the broad themes under consideration included a government-run insurance option designed to foster greater market competitiveness, regulation of insurance industry practices, including prohibitions on preexisting exclusions, an expansion of Medicaid to cover families at higher levels of income than are currently allowed, possible expansions of Medicare to younger recipients, limits on public funding for abortion services to those who received insurance subsidies, a requirement that most employers cover their employees' health insurance premiums, and an individual mandate to purchase or otherwise obtain (usually through an employer) insurance with government subsidies available for low- to moderate-income families and individuals. The bills also contained many other less prominent provisions, including a range of pilot projects designed to explore efficiency-enhancing changes in delivery and payment systems.[20] Funding for new or expanded provisions would come from a combination of general revenues, new taxes on high-end insurance plans (the so-called Cadillac insurance plans, many of which had been hard-won by labor unions through collective bargaining over the years), taxes on elective surgeries, and savings wrung from hoped-for greater efficiencies. By late December, separate House and Senate versions of the legislation won approval in their respective chambers, with estimated 10-year costs of $1.2 trillion for the House version and $871 billion for that of the Senate. Democratic leaders had, with considerable finesse, managed to corral just enough votes to avoid a promised Republican filibuster.[21]

The Obama administration's early urging to pass a bill prior to the August 2009 recess had anticipated rising opposition if the legislative struggle became protracted. This lesson had been learned the hard way in the 1990s, as the Clinton plan lost support during the lengthy delay in sending a bill to Congress, an interim during which White House opponents enjoyed ample time to sow doubts. Congress's August recess, during which members met with constituents in numerous town hall gatherings, provided critics venues to express—literally to scream, in many cases—serious reservations about the pending bills. As complicated negotiations toward cross-chamber reconciliation stretched out through January, the Democrats clung tenuously to their 60-vote, filibuster-proof majority. The anxiety over not sending the president a bill to sign by August had been bad enough. Now Democrats had to acknowledge the renewed difficulty of passing a major bill during an election year, and while November was still a long way off, a special election for a U.S. Senate seat in Massachusetts was not. That balloting would take place on January 19. In the balance hung a vote needed to forestall a Republican filibuster that, if sustained, would likely terminate the Democratic push for passage of a significant bill. The special election produced a Republican victory, and in the short term dashed Democratic hopes for comprehensive reform.

Beyond significant soul-searching about how a Republican could beat a Democrat in liberal Massachusetts, Democrats pondered their next legislative move. None of the options looked promising. The House seemed unlikely to adopt the Senate version of the bill. Senate Democrats seemed unwilling to use an aggressive parliamentary move to outflank the filibuster procedure by hitching a health bill to a budget measure that cannot be filibustered. Some wondered whether one or both of Maine's moderate Republican senators might cooperate. They both indicated potential interest in doing so.[22] However, their suggestion that success will come through the crafting of a consensus bill was predicated on the idea that some significant number of congressional Republicans wanted to seek consensus to move a bill forward. The idea of breaking up the two chambers' large bills and passing them one at a time as smaller bills received some attention but inspired little passion. This piecemeal approach also raised concerns about whether the individual components of reform could be individually engineered to work successfully in concert as a whole. Given the fact that the GOP did not introduce its own alternative bill, and that Republicans largely stayed away from negotiations over the proposals that did progress, and given the declared strategy of obstruction by many of their allies, one could be forgiven for concluding that to seek bipartisanship was a fool's errand in the environment prevailing in early 2010.

WHERE DO WE GO FROM HERE?

Comprehensive policy reform is hard to achieve. Significantly changing government's role in the healthcare sector, an area that accounts for approximately one-seventh of the nation's economy, is especially so. The epigram from Sven Steinmo and Jon Watts that opens this chapter points to incompetent institutions as the reason. This book has argued that they are partially correct. The rest of the story, of course, has to do with Americans' attitudes about their medical providers, the role of government, and people's fears of losing whatever health security they have now. While the debate over institutional versus attitudinal explanations of the difficulty of health reform seems likely to remain vibrant, so too do calls for policy reform itself. Americans have been on the cusp of sweeping health reform before. We will be here again, because issues this big do not tend to fade away.

Bringing this final chapter to an end during a time of lively policy debate has been a challenge. Regardless of where the 2010 debate leads the United States, several themes seem quite likely to persist. A discussion of some possible solutions to the problems surrounding cost of, quality of, and access to health services should shed light on future directions and would seem useful. The remainder of this chapter briefly discusses several of these possible solutions and explores how some of them found their way into healthcare legislation recently under consideration. Whether these provisions make their way into federal legislation in the near term, these are ideas that have secured sufficient purchase in the minds of policy makers that they are likely to persist as part of the healthcare debate.

*   *   *   *

Before moving into the substantive proposals, considering the language of healthcare reform may be helpful. Each time Congress grapples with health legislation, one of the obstacles is a pandemonium over vocabulary. Fear-mongering about socialized medicine has evolved into the language of government takeovers and cold-hearted bureaucracies. Opponents of progressive reform have long hurled these terms in their successful efforts to stunt further government involvement, suggesting that national health insurance would necessarily turn all medical professionals into government employees who would lack incentives to provide the best possible care and medical innovations. It may be useful to distinguish here between socialized healthcare financing, such as Medicare, and socialized medicine, in which doctors and other medical professionals work for government. The United States has practiced the former for decades without sliding into the latter. On the other hand, supporters of progressive health reforms have tended to minimize the import of creating new individual entitlements when they advocate program expansion. Discussion of the cost of a particular added benefit under Medicare tends to overshadow the fact that this is a program that in 2009 cost taxpayers nearly $0.5 trillion. This level of spending was not achieved overnight. Rather, it resulted from many gradual expansions, each of which might be discussed as only a modest increase. Honest discussions of healthcare programming will need to own up to these realities.

The other matter that may or may not be settled anytime soon has been a recurrent theme in these chapters. The market analogy makes, or unmakes, the logic of any particular reform proposal. In part because we are conflicted on this point, decisive solutions have eluded us. Those who see medical purchases as marketlike tend toward financial incentives for conservative and utility-maximizing behavior, but they also tend to downplay the importance of universal provision regardless of ability to pay and the human consequences of noncoverage. Liberals, on the other hand, tend to ignore evidence that to some significant degree, nonpoor people consume health services in ways that partially (but note, *only* partially) reflect marketlike choices. There likely is no objectively determinable ideal level of consumption, but that should not mean that the target should be an ever-rising one, unless we find less painful ways to pay for it. At the very least, all concerned should acknowledge both the power and the limits of market analogies. As healthcare economist Katherine Swartz notes, in conventional markets "the price of a half-gallon of milk or a sweater does not depend on who buys it."[23] With healthcare purchasing, it does. Age, group or individual status, one's health, and many other factors affect the price of services and insurance. Similarly, ability to pay predicts neither high nor low levels of consumption. Policy solutions must acknowledge the selective application of market mechanisms in the health sector. Politicians, who tend to be more enamored of market analogies in health care, may experience more difficulty breaking free of this perspective than will average Americans, given the apparent "pan-ideological consensus in favor of markets [that] has been forged among the Washington elite, . . . [a] position [that] is neither well recognized nor broadly supported outside of the Beltway."[24] Vocabulary matters because of its generative power vis-à-vis ideas, which in turn frame our policy discussions. Discussion of several ideas that are likely to be part of solutions in the near term follows.

Expand Public Programs That Emphasize Basic Health Services

Investing in broader public programs pays handsome dividends. With the growth of public health efforts during the first half of the twentieth century, longevity in the United States rose dramatically, from an average life expectancy of 45 years in 1900 to one of 65 years half a century later. High-tech medicine, on the other hand, appears to have contributed only very slightly to longevity. Cross-nationally, the largest differences in life expectancy are not explained by the widespread practice of high-tech medicine, rather by the presence of well-developed basic public health programs.[25] Public programs may be one way to reach that level of basic service, especially for those who cannot afford to purchase private insurances.

Public health programs are often perceived as drags on government budgets or overly large bureaucracies. While some of them, particularly Medicare and Medicaid, have become very expensive, they also facilitate coverage with relatively little overhead cost. Medicare, for example, involves administrative costs of approximately 3 percent of total expenditures. Compare this to some 25¢ on the dollar for the average private plan. Medicare has also experienced a lower rate of inflation over the past 30 years than have private plans.[26] Medicare expenditures increased an average of 8.9 percent annually from 1970 to 2004, compared to private health insurance premiums that have increased by an average annual rate of 9.9 percent over this period.[27] There may be reasons to resist expanded public programs, but the efficiency of these programs certainly makes them appealing. In this spirit, Congress expanded SCHIP in early 2009, a move that covered an estimated 4,000,000 more children, beyond the 6,000,000 children already included. Practical-minded advocates of larger government programs, such as California Democrat Henry Waxman, have pursued this strategy with significant, albeit gradual, success.

Critics of Medicare will point out that because the Department of Health and Human Services (HSS) dedicates so few resources to payment oversight (it actually employs about 1,500 people in its inspector general's office), fraud runs rampant, costing taxpayers billions of dollars that would not be spent, or wasted, under the watchful eyes of private insurers. Accurate estimates of the extent of Medicare fraud are difficult to obtain, but HHS has assessed improper payments to amount to between 7 and 14 percent of all reimbursements.[28] The agency recovered an average of $1 billion annually from 2006 to 2008 in improper payments under Medicare.[29] While fraud may be more pervasive in Medicare than in the private market, it remains a lesser price to pay than the staggering overhead costs of private insurers.

Move Away from Fee-for-Service

Paying medical providers for each service they perform has been the standard model in American medicine since the beginning. The justification hinges on the idea that doctors, like other skilled service providers, should be paid for each task they perform. Performing more time-consuming or complex tasks should earn the provider more money. However, the incentive this creates for providers to perform many tasks, some of which serve no therapeutic purpose, is powerful. Overutilization, in addition to the legitimate concerns it raises about exposing patients to unnecessary risks, is a major source of medical inflation.

Thinking differently about how to pay providers has led to the idea of pay-for-performance. Under variations of this, providers are paid for treating a patient with a particular diagnosis and are paid partly in accordance with health outcomes. Here the key incentive is to produce a quality outcome rather than to perform an abundance of services. While pay-for-performance seems intuitively better than fee-for-service, empirical evidence on its efficiency is scant.[30] Some will object that paying doctors in relation to outcomes places them at the mercy of the compliance of their patients. Excellent advice from a physician might not end up being financially rewarded by public programs or HMOs if the patient disregards that advice and remains sick.

Despite the early state of knowledge about pay-for-performance, the staff at the Centers for Medicare and Medicaid Services believes this idea has merit. Beginning in 2005 they offered a limited number of grants to physician practices that delivered quality services to Medicare recipients at a lower per capita cost than other medical practices in the area. Dartmouth-Hitchcock Medical Center in New Hampshire met the goal in 2006–2007 and received a $6.7 million for its accomplishments.[31] Whether this idea will both produce financial savings and preserve quality of care remains an open question, but most healthcare policy experts believe the old fee-for-service model should be discarded. In an autumn 2008 survey by the Commonwealth Fund, 69 percent of experts reported that they believe fee-for-service is "not effective," and another 22 percent called it only "somewhat effective."[32] Almost certainly, further incentives toward pay-for-performance will be part of public programs in the foreseeable future.

Comparative Effectiveness

Another approach to thinking about quality over quantity emphasizes evidence-based treatments instead of encouraging medical providers to use a combination of their expertise and their intuition. Studies in comparative effectiveness attempt to empirically determine the best treatment for a given diagnosis. That information can then be used in at least two ways. A soft response is to inform physicians of the comparative effectiveness of various treatments for a given illness and hope that they will employ these best practices with patients. A more hard-hitting response might involve Medicare or Medicaid, or conceivably private insurers, paying only for treatments that rank high in effectiveness for a given diagnosis and withholding payment for any other course of treatment.

Comparative effectiveness will involve its own controversies. In the future, will this practice shackle providers into practicing cookbook medicine to such an extent that it stunts innovation? Will doctors lie to insurance companies about diagnoses in order to buy themselves latitude regarding treatments? These concerns aside, members of Congress believed in its potential enough to have created the Agency for Health Care Policy and Research in 1989. The agency was charged in part to develop suggested treatment standards. In 1996 the AMA endorsed the idea of comparative effectiveness, a turnaround for the organization whose members had previously opposed it. In 2000 this federal office that was renamed the Agency for Healthcare Research and Quality used part of its $200 million budget to fund projects at several research centers and hospitals toward further developing suggested treatment guidelines.[33] Legislation pending in Congress in early 2010 provides funds for studies in comparative effectiveness but would not require doctors to employ the suggested treatments.

Support for comparative effectiveness comes, for instance, in the form of a study that found that among patients with stable coronary artery disease, those who received a stint in addition to drug treatment had better blood flow initially, but over time the differences between these patients and those who received only drug treatments diminished significantly. Their five-year survival rates were not significantly different.[34] In the late 1980s Dr. John Wennberg compared rates of various types of treatments and outcomes of those treatments that were observed in New Haven and Boston during 1982. He found that patients in New Haven were twice as likely to undergo a coronary bypass operation as those in Boston but that patients in Boston were much more likely to have their hips or knees replaced. New Haven residents were much more likely to undergo back operations and hysterectomies.[35] These differences suggest an almost random pattern to treatment, a pattern that ends up being wasteful and likely not as therapeutic as it should be. This is certainly not a pattern that is informed by reliable insights of comparative effectiveness.

The need for more uniform approaches to treatment speaks not only to the quality of treatment but to its cost as well. A recent examination of Medicare expenditures in McAllen, Texas, found that per capita costs are almost

twice the national average, nearly $15,000 per person in 2006. This differ-
ence does not seem to be explained by a high cost of living in the area or by
higher rates of sickness among residents. Rather, from all appearances the
problem is overutilization by doctors. Patients in McAllen tended to receive
more of just about every kind of service: more diagnostics, more hospital
treatment, more surgery, more home health care. This reinforces the adage in
the trade that the most expensive piece of medical equipment around is the doctor's pen. According to surgeon and health commentator Atul Gawande, "as a
rule, hospital executives don't own the pen caps. Doctors do."[36]

Arguments will ensue over the proper locus of studies into comparative
effectiveness. First, looking to the private sector means relying on companies
that may lack financial incentives to conduct thorough-going analyses, as
some of those analyses are going to show competitors' products to be superior. Second, private firms will have an incentive to selectively withhold their
findings or to charge for their dissemination, something that government
would presumably not do. Achieving this public good via private channels
may not work well. On the other hand, critics of government bureaucracy
will almost certainly pounce on the idea of government bureaucrats—
whether they are medical doctors or not—telling physicians what treatments
can or cannot be reimbursed under Medicaid and Medicare.

An Individual Mandate

In 2006 Massachusetts adopted the nation's first individual mandate.
It requires state residents to secure health insurance through their employer,
from the commonwealth's Medicaid program (provided they have sufficiently
low income), from a publicly subsidized insurance program (the Commonwealth Care Health Insurance Program, available to persons earning less than
300 percent of the federal poverty level), or directly from a private insurer.
In the absence of a hardship waiver, individuals who do not carry insurance
face a fine.[37] As of early 2010, no other state has followed Massachusetts'
lead, though law makers in California considered it.

The arguments for an individual mandate usually include the elimination
of cost shifting, assurance that people get the preventative services that help
avoid more serious conditions later, and that by pushing more consumers
into the market, insurance premiums will fall. Problems include the cost to
individuals and the difficulty of enforcement. Just as states typically require
motorists to carry insurance, a significant minority of drivers go without. Further, forcing people to purchase insurance does not directly enhance their
ability to do so. Massachusetts has in place various mechanisms to help, but
for people above the poverty line, this remains a burden. (Massachusetts

residents below the poverty line can get insurance through the state at no cost.) Many conservatives and libertarians dislike an individual mandate because it stands at odds with a free market.[38] Many liberals dislike the idea because, for those persons who cannot get insurance from the state, this represents a forced transaction with a private company.[39] Translation: a bonanza for private insurers. Further, because less expensive policies often carry high deductibles, having insurance does not equate to having access to needed services.

Insurance companies will likely enter negotiations with legislatures suggesting they will reduce premiums in exchange for not opposing healthcare legislation that includes both industry regulation and an individual mandate. They see more paying customers as part of the deal. A variety of politicians, including Barack Obama, have supported an individual mandate, and polls have found majority support among the public for the idea. Surveys by NBC/*Wall Street Journal*, CBS/*New York Times*, and Democracy Corps during June 2009 revealed that majorities or pluralities favor an individual mandate, so long as government assistance is available for those who might struggle to purchase insurance. Typical of the findings were those from a question by CBS/*New York Times*: "As long as the federal government provides financial help to those who cannot afford health insurance, do you think the federal government should or should not require all Americans to have health insurance?" Forty-eight percent said it should, compared to 38 percent who said it should not. Fourteen percent were undecided.[40] As details evolve into legislative specifics, support for and opposition to an individual mandate can be expected to polarize.

A Public Insurance Option

In an effort to create an insurance option for low-income people, liberal Democrats advanced the idea in early 2009 of the federal government as vendor of health insurance to compete with private plans. The Senate was less disposed to this idea than the House of Representatives. Proponents saw this as a way to fill a gap and possibly to provide affordable coverage. Viewed by opponents as the entering wedge toward a single-payer insurance system, the public option quickly became recognized as one of the more hard-to-sell principles of the Obama administration. Robert Moffit at the Heritage Foundation dismissed the administration's idea of the government both regulating and selling insurance as a case of it attempting to be both "umpire and player."[41] In addition to opposition from congressional conservatives, the insurance industry and much of the small business community have opposed the public option. The exception to this came from the Main Street Alliance, a group of some 5,000 small business owners. However, that organization's spring 2009 announcement of support did little, if anything to buoy the idea.[42]

Anathema to nearly all Republicans and controversial enough to give many moderate Democrats pause, the public option provided a target for conservative and antigovernment critics during the summer of 2009. In an effort to defuse this line of criticism, the White House signaled on August 16 that the president viewed the public option as desirable but not essential. Instead, the administration announced its support for federal seed money to build a network of nonprofit entities, perhaps along the lines of Blue Cross and Blue Shield, that would sell insurance at reasonable prices. The goal, to hear administration officials put it, was to find ways to cover all Americans and to reform insurance law to further protect consumers from discrimination based on their health condition. Liberals intent on pushing for a public insurance option responded with pleas for the president to not abandon them, though once a president signals his unwillingness to fight for a controversial idea, the chances of it becoming law become long indeed.

*   *   *   *

Step-by-step reforms have certainly brought about some useful changes over the past few decades, but this approach has also allowed the costs of Medicare, Medicaid, and private insurance to rise to levels previously unimagined and which are unarguably burdensome on the nation's economy. Plans for sweeping changes to healthcare delivery and financing often represent some very sophisticated thinking by smart and well-intentioned people, but those plans often call for leaps of faith that involve political vulnerabilities fostered by the attitudinal and institutional constraints discussed here. Appeals to moral suasion are only so powerful. President Obama often invoked the language of the absolute imperative of major reform, telling audiences that "the status quo is untenable," and "everybody understands we can't keep doing what we are doing. It is bankrupting families. . . . It is bankrupting businesses. . . . And it's bankrupting our government at the state and federal levels. So we know things are going to change."[43] Even lobbyists for the insurance industry, the arch-enemy as far as many liberals are concerned, acknowledge that the status quo is no longer viable. Dan Danner—lobbyist for the National Federation of Independent Businesses, primarily a small business group with strong GOP ties—in the summer of 2009 referred to how much the landscape has changed since the 1990s. "The difference is that 15 years ago, our members felt that the status quo was better than what was being proposed. . . . This time the status quo isn't acceptable."[44] The trouble is, saying this does not make it so. Incremental change at the margins seems the most likely outcome in the near term. But even multiple episodes of minor reform do not necessarily build coherently and constructively one upon the other, thus prudent steps do not necessarily sum to a fundamental redress for the host of problems that have taken roughly a century to develop. Incrementalism does not appear to likely produce a comprehensive healthcare system, but it seems to be the most realistic alternative Americans have.

NOTES

1. Rothman 1994, p. 14.
2. Steinmo and Watts 1995, p. 330.
3. Feldman and Steenbergen 2001; Shaw 2009/2010.
4. Dick Armey and Newt Gingrich, "The Welfarization of Health Care," *National Review*, February 7, 1994, p. 53.
5. White 1995, p. 375.
6. "Thinking now about national priorities, how important is the goal of Congress and the President guaranteeing universal health insurance for every American by the end of 2009? . . . The most important priority, one of the top 2–3 priorities, an important goal, but not a top priority, not important at all?" (Survey by Ipsos-Public Affairs, April 30–May 3, 2009, N = 1,004)
7. "What about reforming health care? Should this be one of their top priorities, very important but not a top priority, somewhat important, or not that important?" (Survey by Princeton Survey Research Associates International, July 7–14, 2009, N = 1,205)
8. Roemer 1945, p. 163.
9. Ibid., p. 159.
10. Kaiser Family Foundation 2007, pp. 7–8.
11. 2005 report of the Social Security Trustees (available online at www.socialsecurity.gov).
12. Jost 2007, p. 10.
13. Bara Vaida, "Super Bowl Moment," *National Journal*, June 13, 2009, p. 22.
14. Frank Luntz, "The Language of Healthcare, 2009" (available online at http://wonkroom.thinkprogress.org/wp-content/uploads/2009/05/frank-luntz-the-language-of-healthcare-20091.pdf; accessed January 22, 2010).
15. Kristol memo, available online at http:/www.scribd.com/doc/12926608/William-Kristols-1993-Memo-Defeating-President-Clintons-Health-Care-Proposal?autodown=pdf (accessed May 22, 2009).
16. Frank Luntz, "The Language of Healthcare, 2009."
17. Ibid., p. 1 (emphasis in original).
18. Paul West, "GOP Rides Wave of Ire," *The Baltimore Sun*, August 16, 2009, p. 1A.
19. Andy Zajac, "Insurance Option Not Essential," *Chicago Tribune*, August 17, 2009, p. 10.
20. Atul Gawande, "Testing, Testing," *The New Yorker*, vol. 85, #41, December 14, 2009, pp. 34–41.

21. James Oliphant, "After Passing 2 Health Bills, Hill Must Now Build Bridge," *Chicago Tribune*, December 27, 2009, Nation & World section, p. 1.

22. David Sharpe, "Snow Still Willing to Cooperate with Democrats on Health Bill," *Boston Globe* (online version, Boston.com), January 23, 2010.

23. Swartz 2006, p. 60.

24. Schlesinger 2005, p. 122.

25. Engel 2006, p. 94.

26. Barlett and Steele 2004, p. 238.

27. Jost 2007, p. 10.

28. Becker et al. 2005, p. 190.

29. Testimony of Daniel Levinson, HHS Inspector General, before the House Energy and Commerce Committee, Subcommittee on Health, June 25, 2009 (available online at www.oig.hhs.gov; accessed July 8, 2009).

30. See Rosenthal 2006.

31. *Dartmouth Medicine*, Winter 2008 (available online at www.dartmed .dartmouth.edu; accessed July 8, 2009).

32. Stremikis et al. 2008, p. 2.

33. Coombs 2005, p. 252.

34. Congressional Budget Office, "Research on the Comparative Effectiveness of Medical Treatments" (December 2007, publication # 2975), p. 4. For a counterpoint, see Helen Evans, "Comparative Effectiveness in Health Care Reform: Lessons from Abroad," February 24, 2009 (available online at heritage.org; accessed July 9, 2009).

35. Joseph Califano, "The Health-Care Chaos," *New York Times*, March 20, 1988, section 6, p. 44.

36. Gawande, "Testing, Testing," p. 40.

37. Massachusetts Trial Court Law Libraries, "Health Care Access Law: Frequently Asked Questions" (available online at www.lawlib.state.ma.us/healthinsurance/html; accessed October 1, 2007).

38. See Michael Tanner, "Individual Mandates for Health Insurance: Slippery Slope to National Health Care," April 5, 2006 (available online at www.cato.org; accessed July 9, 2009).

39. See "An Individual Mandate for Health Insurance: Unwise, Unwarranted, Unworkable," December 6, 2006 (available online at www.newamerica.net; accessed July 9, 2009).

40. CBS/*New York Times* poll, June 12–16, 2009 (N = 895 adults).

41. Robert Moffit and Nina Owcharenko, "The Obama Health Care Plan: More Power to Washington" (available online at www.heritage.org; accessed April 29, 2009).

42. Vaida, "Super Bowl Moment," p. 27.

43. Comments available at www.cnn.com/2009/politics/06/25/health.care/index.html (accessed June 25, 2009).

44. Vaida, "Super Bowl Moment," p. 22.

Appendix 1

Timeline of Significant Events in American Health Care

1798	Congress enacts the Relief of Sick and Disabled Seamen Act, creating the Marine Hospital Fund.
1847	The American Medical Association is founded largely in response to the spread of unorthodox medical practitioners.
1850s	Effective anesthesia is invented, allowing for safer, less painful surgical procedures.
1860s	Physicians develop the germ theory of infection.
1874	Andrew Still begins the practice of osteopathy in the United States focusing on more holistic medicine.
1878	Congress creates the Marine Hospital Service.
1883	Harvey Washington Wiley is appointed chief chemist at the U.S. Department of Agriculture's Division of Chemistry and is given authority to investigate fraudulent medicines.
1897	Students at the Kirksville, Missouri, American School of Osteopathy form the American Association for the Advancement of Osteopathy, renamed the American Osteopathic Association in 1901.
	Daniel Palmer establishes the Palmer School for Cure, now known as the Palmer College of Chiropractic, in Davenport, Iowa.
1898	The American Hospital Association is founded.
Late 1890s	The X-ray is developed to examine patients.

1905	Samuel Hopkins authors an article in *Colliers* magazine titled "The Great American Fraud," which calls attention to the problems of nostrums and snake oil remedies.
1906	Members of the Palmer School of Chiropractic organize the Universal Chiropractors Association in order to defend chiropractors from persecution.
1910	The publication of the Flexner Report marks a turning point in American medical education.
1911	Britain adopts the National Insurance Act, which becomes a common reference point for American progressives calling for similar action in the United States.
1912	The American Association for Labor Legislation begins a campaign to advocate the adoption of compulsory health insurance laws in the states and at the federal level.
	Congress creates the United States Children's Bureau within the Department of Commerce and Labor in response to concern over child labor practices.
1916	The American Association for Labor Legislation's compulsory healthcare bill is introduced in the New York State Senate.
1921	Congress passes the Sheppard-Towner Act, creating grant programs for maternal and child health and hygiene.
1927	The USDA's Bureau of Chemistry is transformed into the Food, Drug, and Insecticide Organization—this later becomes the Food and Drug Administration in 1930. The Sheppard-Towner Act expires.
1929	Baylor University Hospital launches a nonprofit health insurance pool, marking the beginning of Blue Cross.
1935	Healthcare provisions are stripped from the administration's bill that becomes the Social Security Act out of worry by President Roosevelt that their inclusion might undermine support for retirement pensions.
1938	Industrialist Henry J. Kaiser forms the first prepaid health insurance plan, an early health maintenance organization; this plan is formalized as a separate corporation, Kaiser Permanente, in 1942.
1943	The first of many versions of the Wagner-Murray-Dingell bill is introduced in Congress.
1945	President Truman announces support for compulsory health insurance.
1948	Congress passes the Hill-Burton Act to fund the construction of hospitals and clinics.
1955	Congress creates the Indian Health Service, which takes over services for American Indian and Alaska Native people from the Bureau of Indian Affairs.

1957	Representative Aimee Forand introduces a bill to cover Social Security recipients under what would become Medicare in 1965.
1960	The Kerr-Mills program, precursor to Medicaid, is enacted.
	Americans spend 5.3 percent of Gross Domestic Product on health care.
1963	The American Chiropractic Association is founded.
1965	Medicare and Medicaid are enacted.
1969	The Kerr-Mills program ends.
1970	Senator Edward Kennedy introduces a bill to create the Health Security Act, a single-payer system.
	Minnesota physician Paul Ellwood and his study group coin the term "health maintenance organization."
	Americans spend 7.3 percent of GDP on health care.
1973	The Health Maintenance Organization Assistance Act becomes law, providing a legal framework and federal grants to create modern HMOs.
1974	President Nixon presents his Comprehensive Health Insurance bill, which includes an employer mandate and voluntary employee participation. The bill does not pass Congress.
1979	Senator Edward Kennedy introduces a bill to create the Health Care for All Americans Act.
1980	Americans spend 9.2 percent of GDP on health care.
1981	President Reagan proposes that the federal government could assume responsibility for Medicaid in exchange for the states taking over welfare; the administration found no willing congressional sponsors for such a bill.
1982	Congress enacts the Tax Equity and Financial Responsibility Act, allowing managed care to expand into the Medicare program.
1983	Medicare's Prospective Payment System changes the way most hospitals are paid for most services, based no longer on reasonable charges but rather on a prospective determination of what a given illness episode should cost to treat. This change saves taxpayers billions of dollars each year.
1988	Congress enacts a catastrophic coverage component to Medicare.
1989	In the face of withering criticism from seniors who are angry over higher premiums, Congress repeals the catastrophic coverage component of Medicare.
1990	Americans spend 12.2 percent of GDP on health care.

1991   Harris Wofford successfully campaigns on health care, winning a U.S. Senate race from Pennsylvania. His victory catalyzes health care as an important political issue, particularly for Democrats.

1993   President Clinton launches his effort to create a government-organized system of managed competition.

1994   Congressional willingness to consider the Clinton plan collapses.

1996   Congress creates a pilot program for a limited number of tax-sheltered medical savings accounts; this program is enlarged significantly in 2003.

1997   Congress enacts the State Children's Health Insurance Program, an optional federal-state shared program to assist children in low- to moderate-income families.

2003   Congress enacts a prescription drug benefit under Medicare and expands tax-sheltered health savings accounts.

2006   Americans spend 16 percent of GDP on health care.

2009   The Obama administration works with Congress to reform healthcare financing and insurance regulation.

2010   Popular and congressional support fades for a sweeping healthcare reform effort.

Appendix 2

Annotated List of Further Readings: Selected Topics

HISTORY OF MEDICINE

Paul Starr. *The Social Transformation of American Medicine: The Rise of a Sovereign Profession and the Making of a Vast Industry.* New York: Basic Books, 1982. A Pulitzer Prize–winning and widely read classic on the emergence of the modern medical establishment.

Morris Fishbein. *A History of the American Medical Association.* Philadelphia: W. B. Saunders Company, 1947. A history of the nation's largest medical society and lobbying group, written by a one-time editor of the *Journal of the American Medical Association.*

James H. Cassedy. *Medicine in America: A Short History.* Baltimore: The Johns Hopkins University Press, 1991. A brief history of medicine from early America up through the 1980s.

Richard Shryock. *Medical Licensing in America, 1650–1965.* Baltimore: The Johns Hopkins University Press, 1967. An excellent history of medical licensing.

EARLY TO MID-TWENTIETH CENTURY

Ronald Numbers. *Almost Persuaded: American Physicians and Compulsory Health Insurance, 1912–1920.* Baltimore: The Johns Hopkins University Press, 1978. A detailed and highly readable account of the AMA's initial support for but later opposition to national health insurance.

Daniel Hirshfield. *The Lost Reform: The Campaign for Compulsory Health Insurance in the United States from 1932 to 1943.* Cambridge, MA: Harvard University Press,

1970. A thoughtful and detailed account of the failure of New Deal–era health reform advocates to incorporate health insurance under the Social Security Act.

Monte Poen, *Harry S. Truman Versus the Medical Lobby: The Genesis of Medicare.* Columbia: University of Missouri Press, 1979. Probably the best treatment of Truman's struggle with the AMA over compulsory health insurance legislation.

THE CREATION OF MEDICARE AND MEDICAID

Theodore Marmor. *The Politics of Medicare.* Hawthorne, NY: Aldine De Gruyter, 1970. The best single account of the creation of Medicare. Updated in a second edition in 2000.

Robert Stevens and Rosemary Stevens. *Welfare Medicine in America: A Case Study of Medicaid.* New York: Free Press, 1974. A comprehensive treatment of the political struggle to expand public charity health programs into the Medicaid program in 1965 with an early assessment of its results.

RECENT DEVELOPMENTS IN HEALTHCARE POLITICS

Randy Shilts. *And the Band Played On: Politics, People, and the AIDS Epidemic.* New York: Penguin Books, 1987. A highly readable, frank, and at times raw assessment of the federal government's slow response to the emergence of AIDS in the 1980s.

Jonathan Oberlander. *The Political Life of Medicare.* Chicago: University of Chicago Press, 2003. A very good treatment of some of the recent political and financial challenges facing Medicare.

Alain Enthoven. *Health Plan: The Only Practical Solution to the Soaring Cost of Medical Care*, 1980. Written by the principal architect of the managed competition model, this book articulates many of the ideas that would later make up the Clinton plan.

Jacob Hacker. *The Road to Nowhere: The Genesis of President Clinton's Plan for Health Security.* Princeton, NJ: Princeton University Press, 1997. A detailed examination of the development of the Clinton plan.

ARGUMENTS FOR AND AGAINST NATIONAL HEALTH INSURANCE

Jill Quadagno. *One Nation Uninsured: Why the U.S. Has No National Health Insurance.* New York: Oxford University Press, 2005. A liberal assessment of the historic opposition to national health insurance that draws heavily on many oral histories from key political actors.

Philip Funigiello. *Chronic Politics: Health Care Security from FDR to George W. Bush.* Lawrence: University Press of Kansas, 2005. Documents the political conflicts over national health policy and mines archives of the papers of political actors along the way.

Arnold Relman. *A Second Opinion: Rescuing America's Health Care*. New York: Public Affairs (Perseus), 2007. A critical examination of modern medical financing and a call for a single-payer system, written by a Harvard Medical School professor and former editor of the *New England Journal of Medicine*.

Richard Epstein. *Mortal Peril: Our Inalienable Right to Health Care?* Reading, MA: Addison-Wesley Publishers, 1997. A strident challenge to the idea of public health insurance, and a defense for treating health care as an economic market.

Timothy Jost. *Health Care at Risk: A Critique of the Consumer-Driven Movement*. Durham, NC: Duke University Press, 2007. A penetrating critique of the consumer-driven healthcare movement.

ONLINE RESOURCES

American Medical Association (www.ama-assn.org)—The nation's largest medical society and a key player in healthcare politics since the early twentieth century. The Web site includes history; coverage of numerous current issues; resources for physicians, researchers, and the general public.

The Commonwealth Fund (www.commonwealthfund.org)—A private foundation that pursues health policy education. It publishes reports and data on the U.S. and international healthcare outcomes and the U.S. politics of health care.

The Milbank Memorial Fund (www.milbank.org)—A private foundation that distributes information on health and population issues and has published a journal, *The Milbank Quarterly: A Multidisciplinary Journal of Population Health and Health Policy*, for more than 80 years.

Henry J. Kaiser Family Foundation (www.kkf.org)—A private foundation that produces educational materials on a wide variety of U.S. healthcare issues. The foundation also regularly partners with National Public Radio and the Harvard School of Public Health to conduct public opinion polling on healthcare topics.

America's Health Insurance Plans (www.ahip.org)—An association of approximately 1,300 health insurance companies. Their Web site includes information for policy advocates, insurance companies, and consumers.

Bibliography

Altmeyer, Arthur. *The Formative Years of Social Security.* Madison: University of Wisconsin Press, 1966.

Anderson, Odin. *Health Services in the United States: A Growth Enterprise since 1875.* Ann Arbor, MI: Health Administration Press, 1985.

Anderson, G., and W. Scanlon. "Medicaid Payment Policy and the Boren Amendment," pp. 82–94 in D. Rowland, J. Feder, and A. Salganicoff (eds.), *Medicaid Financing Crisis: Balancing Responsibilities, Priorities and Dollars.* American Association for the Advancement of Science, 1993.

Arney, William. *Power and the Profession of Obstetrics.* Chicago: University of Chicago Press, 1982.

Arrow, Kenneth. "Uncertainty and the Welfare Economics of Medical Care," *American Economic Review* 53 (1963): 941–973.

Balkin, Karen. *Health Care* (Opposing Viewpoints series). Farmington Hills, MI: Greenhaven Press, 2003.

Barlett, Donald, and James Steele. *Critical Condition: How Health Care in America Became Big Business and Bad Medicine.* New York: Doubleday, 2004.

Beck, Andrew. "The Flexner Report and the Standardization of American Medical Education," *The Journal of the American Medical Association* 291 (May 5, 2004): 2139–2140.

Becker, David, Daniel Kessler, and Mark McClellan. "Detecting Medicare Abuse," *Journal of Health Economics* 24 (2005): 189–210.

Billings, John. "Ideals of Medical Education," *Science* 18 (# 439, July 1891): 1–4.

Bremner, Robert. *From the Depths: The Discovery of Poverty in the United States.* New York: New York University Press, 1956.

Brodie, Mollyann, and Robert Blendon. "The Public's Contribution to Congressional Gridlock on Health Care Reform," *Journal of Health Politics, Policy and Law* 20 (#2, summer 1995): 403–410.

Buchanan, James. *The Demand and Supply of Public Goods.* Chicago: Rand McNally, 1968.

Budrys, Grace. *Our Unsystematic Health Care System, 2nd edition.* New York: Rowman & Littlefield Publishers, Inc. 2005.

Burke, Vincent, and Vee Burke. *Nixon's Good Deed: Welfare Reform.* New York: Columbia University Press, 1974.

Burrow, James. *AMA: Voice of American Medicine.* Baltimore: The Johns Hopkins University Press, 1963.

Califano, Jr., Joseph. *Governing America: An Insider's Report from the White House and the Cabinet.* New York: Simon and Schuster, 1981.

Campion, Frank. *The AMA and U.S. Health Policy since 1940.* Chicago: Chicago Review Press, 1984.

Cassedy, James. *Medicine in America: A Short History.* Baltimore: The Johns Hopkins University Press, 1991.

Clinton, Hillary Rodham. *Living History.* New York: Scribner, 2003.

Congressional Research Service. *Medicaid Source Book: Background Data and Analysis: A 1993 Update.* Washington, DC: United States Government Printing Office, 1993.

Conlan, Timothy. *From New Federalism to Devolution: Twenty-Five Years of Intergovernmental Reform.* Washington, DC: Brookings Institution, 1998.

Coombs, Jan Gregorie. *The Rise and Fall of HMOs: An American Health Care Revolution.* Madison: University of Wisconsin Press, 2005.

Coughlin, Teresa, Leighton Ku, and John Holanhan. *Medicaid since 1980: Costs, Coverage, and the Shifting Alliance between the Federal Government and the States.* Washington, DC: The Urban Institute Press, 1994.

Cunningham, Peter. "SCHIP Making Progress: Increased Take-Up Contributes to Coverage Gains," *Health Affairs* 22 (#4, 2003): 163–172.

Derickson, Alan. "The House of Falk: The Paranoid Style in American Health Politics," *American Journal of Public Health* 87 (#11, November 1997): 1836–1843.

DeVries, Raymond, Cecilia Benoit, Edwin Van Teijlingen, and Sirpa Wrede (eds.). *Birth by Design: Pregnancy, Maternity Care, and Midwifery in North America and Europe.* New York: Routledge, 2001.

Diamond, Jared. *Guns, Germs, and Steel: The Fates of Human Societies.* New York: W. W. Norton & Company, 1997.

Duffy, John. *The Sanitarians: A History of American Public Health.* Urbana, IL: University of Illinois Press, 1990.

Ellwood, Paul, and Alain Enthoven. " 'Responsible Choices': The Jackson Hole Group Pan for Health Reform," *Health Affairs* 14 (#2, 1995): 24–39.

Engel, Jonathan. *Poor People's Medicine: Medicaid and American Charity Care since 1965.* Durham, NC: Duke University Press, 2006.

Enthoven, Alain. *Health Plan: The Only Practical Solution to the Soaring Cost of Medical Care*. Reading, MA: Addison-Wesley, 1980.

Epstein, Richard A. *Mortal Peril: Our Inalienable Right to Health Care?* Reading, MA: Addison-Wesley, 1997.

Falkson, Joseph. *HMOs and the Politics of Health System Reform*. Chicago: American Hospital Association, 1980.

Feder, Judith. *Medicare: The Politics of Federal Hospital Insurance*. Lexington, MA: Lexington Books, 1977.

Federal Trade Commission, "Improving Health Care: A Dose of Competition," 2004.

Fein, Rashi. *Medical Care, Medical Costs*. Cambridge, MA: Harvard University Press, 1986.

Feingold, Eugene. *Medicare: Policy and Politics, A Case Study and Policy Analysis*. San Francisco: Chandler Publishing Company, 1966.

Feldman, Stanley, and Marco Steenbergen. "Social Welfare Attitudes and the Humanitarian Sensibility," pp. 366–400 in James Kuklinski (ed.), *Citizens and Politics: Perspectives from Political Psychology*. New York: Cambridge University Press, 2001.

Feldstein, Martin. "The Welfare Loss of Excess Health Insurance," *Journal of Political Economy* 81 (March/April 1973): 251–280.

Ferling, John. *The First of Men: A Life of George Washington*. Knoxville: University of Tennessee Press, 1989.

Fishbein, Morris. *A History of the American Medical Association, 1847–1947*. Philadelphia: W. B. Saunders Co., 1947.

Fox, Daniel. "From Reform to Relativism: A History of Economists and Health Care," *The Milbank Quarterly* 57 (#3, 1979): 297–336.

Funigiello, Philip. *Chronic Politics: Health Care Security from FDR to George W. Bush*. Lawrence: University of Kansas Press, 2005.

Gamble, Vanessa (ed.). *Germs Have No Color Line: Blacks and American Medicine, 1900–1945*. New York: Garland Publishers, 1988.

Gawande, Atul. "The Cost Conundrum," *The New Yorker* (June 1, 2009): 36–44.

Goodman, John, and Gerald Musgrave. *Patient Power: Solving America's Health Care Crisis*. Washington, DC: Cato Institute, 1992.

Hacker, Jacob. *The Road to Nowhere: The Genesis of President Clinton's Plan for Health Security*. Princeton, NJ: Princeton University Press, 1997.

Harrington, Charlene. "Medical Ideologies in Conflict," *Medical Care* 13 (#11, November 1975): 905–914.

Harris, Richard. *A Sacred Trust*. New York: The New American Library, 1966.

Herz, Elicia, Chris Peterson, and Evelyne Baumraker. "State Children's Health Insurance Program (SCHIP): A Brief Overview," pp. 99–128 in Mary Ewing (ed.), *State Children's Health Insurance Program*. New York: Nova Science Publishers, 2008.

Herzlinger, Regina E. *Market-Driven Health Care*. Reading, MA: Addison-Wesley, 1997.

———— (ed.). *Consumer-Driven Health Care: Implications for Providers, Payers, and Policymakers*. San Francisco: Jossey-Bass, 2004.

Hiaat, Mark, and Christopher Stockton. "The Impact of the Flexner Report on the Fate of Medical Schools in North America after 1909." *Journal of American Physicians and Surgeons* 8 (#2, summer 2003): 37–40.

Himelfarb, Richard. *Catastrophic Politics: The Rise and Fall of Medicare Catastrophic Coverage*. University Park: The Pennsylvania State University Press, 1995.

Himmelstein, David, Sidney Wolfe, and Steffie Woolhander. "Mangled Competition," *The American Prospect* 13 (spring, 1993): 116.

Hirshfield, Daniel. *The Lost Reform: The Campaign for Compulsory Health Insurance in the United States from 1932 to 1943*. Cambridge, MA: Harvard University Press, 1970.

Hoffman, Beatrix. *The Wages of Sickness: The Politics of Health Insurance in Progressive America*. Chapel Hill: University of North Carolina Press, 2001.

Holahan, John, Marilyn Moon, W. Pete Welch, and Stephen Zuckerman. *Balancing Access, Costs, and Politics: The American Context for Health System Reform*. Washington, DC: The Urban Institute Press, 1991.

Holahan, John, Teresa Coughlin, Leighton Ku, D. Heslam, and C. Winterbottom. "The States' Response to Medicaid Financing Crises: Case Studies Report," a report from the Kaiser Commission on the Future of Medicaid, Baltimore, MD, 1992.

Howell, Joel. *Technology in the Hospital: Transforming Patient Care in the Early Twentieth Century*. Baltimore, MD: The Johns Hopkins University Press, 1995.

Hudson, Robert. "Abraham Flexner in Historical Perspective," pp. 1–18 in Barbara Barzansky and Norman Gevitz (eds.), *Beyond Flexner: Medical Education in the Twentieth Century*. Westport, CT: Greenwood Press, 1992.

Hutchison, Tony. "The Medicaid Budget Bust," *State Legislatures* 17 (June 1991): 10–15.

Hyman, David, and William Kovacic. "Monopoly, Monopsony, and Market Definition: An Antitrust Perspective on Market Concentration among Health Insurers," *Health Affairs* 23 (#6, November/December 2004): 25–28.

Jacobs, Lawrence. *The Health of Nations: Public Opinion and the Making of American and British Health Policy*. Ithaca, NY: Cornell University Press, 1993a.

————. "Health Reform Impasse: The Politics of American Ambivalence toward Government," *Journal of Health Politics, Policy and Law* 18 (#3, fall 1993b): 629–655.

Jacobs, Lawrence, and Robert Y. Shapiro. "Don't Blame the Public for Failed Health Care Reform," *Journal of Health Politics, Policy and Law* 20 (#2, summer 1995): 411–423.

————. *Politicians Don't Pander: Political Manipulation and the Loss of Democratic Responsiveness*. Chicago: University of Chicago Press, 2000.

Jecker, Nancy. "Can an Employer-Based Health Insurance System be Just?" pp. 259–275 in James Morone and Gary Belkin (eds.), *The Politics of Health Care Reform:*

Lessons from the Past, Prospects for the Future. Durham, NC: Duke University Press, 1994.

Johnson, Haynes, and David Broder. *The System: The American Way of Politics at the Breaking Point*. Boston: Little Brown, 1996.

Jost, Timothy. *Health Care at Risk: A Critique of the Consumer-Driven Movement*. Durham, NC: Duke University Press, 2007.

Kaiser Family Foundation. "The Uninsured: A Primer—Key Facts about Americans without Health Insurance." October 2007.

Katz, Michael. *In the Shadow of the Poorhouse: A Social History of Welfare in America, 10th Anniversary Edition*. New York: Basic Books, 1996.

Kenny, Genevieve, and Justin Yee. "SCHIP at a Crossroads: Experiences to Date and Challenges Ahead," *Health Affairs* 26 (#2, March/April 2007): 356–369.

Klein, Jennifer. *For All Those Rights: Business, Labor, and the Shaping of America's Public-Private Welfare State*. Princeton, NJ: Princeton University Press, 2003.

Klepp, Susan. "Malthusian Miseries and the Working Poor in Philadelphia, 1780–1830," pp. 63–92 in Billy Smith (ed.), *Down and Out in Early America*. University Park: Pennsylvania State University Press, 2004.

Kooijman, Jaap. *And the Pursuit of National Health: The Incremental Strategy toward National Health Insurance in the United States*. Atlanta, GA: Rodopi, 1999.

Law, Sylvia. *Blue Cross: What Went Wrong?* New Haven, CT: Yale University Press, 1974.

Lee, R. Alton. *From Snake Oil to Medicine: Pioneering Public Health*. Westport, CT: Praeger, 2007.

Litoff, Judy. *The American Midwife Debate: A Sourcebook on Its Modern Origins*. Westport, CT: Greenwood Press, 1986.

Marmor, Theodore. "A Summer of Discontent: Press Coverage of Murder and Medical Care Reform," *Journal of Health Politics, Policy and Law* 20 (#2, summer 1995): 495–501.

———. *The Politics of Medicare, 2nd edition*. New York: Aldine de Gruyter, 1999.

McCaughey, Elizabeth. "No Exit," *The New Republic* 210 (#6, February 7, 1994): 21–25.

Melhado, Evan. "Economists, Public Provision, and the Market," *Journal of Health Politics, Policy and Law* 23 (#2, April 1998): 215–263.

Morais, Herbert. *The History of the Negro in Medicine*. New York: Publisher's Company, Inc., 1967.

Morantz-Sanchez, Regina. *Sympathy and Science: Women Physicians in American Medicine*. New York: Oxford University Press, 1985.

Morone, James. *The Democratic Wish: Popular Participation and the Limits of American Government*. New York: Basic Books, 1990.

Navarro, Vicente. *The Politics of Health Policy*. New York: Cambridge, 1994.

———. "Why Congress Did Not Enact Health Care Reform," *Journal of Health Care Politics, Policy and Law* 20 (#2, summer 1995): 455–462.

Newhouse, Joseph, and the Insurance Experiment Group. *Free for All? Lessons from the Rand Health Insurance Experiment*. Cambridge, MA: Harvard University Press, 1993.

Numbers, Ronald. *Almost Persuaded: American Physicians and Compulsory Health Insurance, 1912–1920*. Baltimore: The Johns Hopkins University Press, 1978.

Oberlander, Jonathan. *The Political Life of Medicare*. Chicago: University of Chicago Press, 2003.

Oliver, Thomas. "Policy Entrepreneurship in the Social Transformation of Medicine: The Rise of Managed Care and Managed Competition," *Journal of Health Politics, Policy and Law* 49 (2004): 701–733.

Oliver, Thomas, Philip Lee, and Helene Lipton. "A Political History of Medicare and Prescription Drug Coverage," *The Milbank Quarterly* 82 (#2, 2004): 283–354.

Pauly, Mark. *Medical Care at Public Expense: A Study in Applied Welfare Economics*. New York: Praeger, 1971.

———. "The Economics of Moral Hazard: Comment," *American Economic Review* 58 (#3, 1968): 531–537.

Pellegrino, Edmund. "Managed Care at the Bedside: How Do We Look in the Moral Mirror?" *Kennedy Institute of Ethics Journal* 7 (December 1997): 321–330.

Peterson, Mark. "The Health Care Debate: All Heat and No Light," *Journal of Health Politics, Policy and Law* 20 (#2, summer 1995): 425–430.

Pierson, Paul. "The New Politics of the Welfare State," *World Politics* 48(#2): 143–179, 1996.

Poen, Monte. *Harry S. Truman versus the Medical Lobby*. Columbia, MO: University of Missouri Press, 1979.

Quadagno, Jill. "Physician Sovereignty and the Purchasers' Revolt," *Journal of Health Politics, Policy, and Law* 29 (#4, August 2004): 815–834.

———. *One Nation, Uninsured: Why the U.S. Has No National Health Insurance*. New York: Oxford University Press, 2005.

Reagan, Michael. *The Accidental System: Health Care Policy in America*. Boulder, CO: Westview Press. 1999.

Relman, Arnold. *A Second Opinion: Rescuing America's Health Care*. New York: Public Affairs, 2007.

Richardson, James. *The Origin and Development of Group Hospitalization in the United States, 1890–1940*. Columbia, MO: University of Missouri Press, 1945.

Roemer, Milton. "Government's Role in American Medicine—A Brief Historical Survey," *Bulletin of the History of Medicine* 18 (1945): 146–168.

Rorty, James. *American Medicine Mobilizes*. New York: W. W. Norton & Co., 1939.

Rosenberg, Charles. *The Cholera Years: The United States in 1832, 1949, and 1866*. Chicago: University of Chicago Press, 1962.

Rosenthal, Meredith. "How Will Paying for Performance Affect Patient Care?" *Ethics Journal of the American Medical Association* 8 (#3, March 2006): 162–165.

Rothman, David. "A Century of Failure: Class Barriers to Reform," pp. 11–25 in James Morone and Gary Belkin (eds.), *The Politics of Health Care Reform: Lessons from the Past, Prospects for the Future*. Durham, NC: Duke University Press, 1994.

———. *The Discovery of the Asylum: Social Order and Disorder in the New Republic*. Boston: Little, Brown & Company, 1971.

Rubinow, Isaac M. *Standards of Health Insurance*. New York: Henry Holt & Co., 1916.

Savitt, Todd. "Abraham Flexner and the Black Medical Schools," pp. 65–81 in Barbara Barzansky and Norman Gevitz (eds.), *Beyond Flexner: Medical Education in the Twentieth Century*. Westport, CT: Greenwood Press, 1992.

Schlesinger, Mark. "The Dangers of the Market Panacea," pp. 91–134 in James Morone and Lawrence Jacobs (eds.), *Healthy, Wealthy, and Fair: Health Care and the Good Society*. New York: Oxford University Press, 2005.

Shaw, Greg M. *The Welfare Debate*. Westport, CT: Greenwood Press, 2007.

Shaw, Greg M. "Changes in Public Opinion and the American Welfare State," *Political Science Quarterly* 124 (winter 2009/2010): 627–653.

Shryock, Richard. *Medical Licensing in America, 1650–1965*. Baltimore, MD: The Johns Hopkins University Press, 1967.

Skocpol, Theda. *Boomerang: Clinton's Health Security Effort and the Turn against Government in U.S. Politics*. New York: W. W. Norton & Co., 1996.

Smith, David. *Entitlement Politics: Medicare and Medicaid, 1995–2001*. New York: Aldine de Gruyter, 2002.

Somers, Herman, and Anne Somers. *Doctors, Patients, and Health Insurance: The Organization and Financing of Medical Care*. Washington, DC: Brookings Institution, 1961.

Starr, Paul. *The Logic of Health Care Reform*. Knoxville, TN: Whittle Direct Books, 1992.

———. *The Social Transformation of American Medicine: The Rise of a Sovereign Profession and the Making of a Vast Industry*. New York: Basic Books, 1982.

———. "The Undelivered Health System," *The Public Interest* 42 (1976): 66–85.

———. "What Happened to Health Care Reform?" *American Prospect* no. 20 (winter 1995): 20–31.

Steinmo, Sven, and Jon Watts. "It's the Institutions, Stupid! Why Comprehensive National Health Insurance Always Fails in America," *Journal of Health Politics, Policy and Law* 20 (#2, summer 1995): 329–372.

Stevens, Rosemary. *American Medicine and the Public Interest*. New Haven, CT: Yale University Press, 1971.

Stevens, Robert, and Rosemary Stevens. *Welfare Medicine in America: A Case Study in Medicaid*. New York: Macmillan, 1974.

Stone, Deborah. "The Struggle for the Soul of Health Insurance," *Journal of Health Politics, Policy and Law* 18 (#2, summer 1993): 287–317.

Stremikis, Kristof, Stuart Guterman, and Karen Davis. "Health Care Opinion Leaders' Views on Payment System Reform," The Commonwealth Fund (publication number 1189, vol. 13, November 2008, available online at www.commonwealthfund.org, accessed March 4, 2009).

Sundquist, James. *Politics and Policy: The Eisenhower, Kennedy, and Johnson Years*. Washington, DC: Brookings Institution, 1968.

Swartz, Katherine. *Reinsuring Health: Why More Middle-Class People Are Uninsured and What Government Can Do*. New York: Russell Sage Foundation, 2006.

Tanenbaum, Sandra. "Medicaid Eligibility Policy in the 1980s: Medical Utilitarianism and the 'Deserving' Poor," *Journal of Health Politics, Policy and Law* 20 (#4, winter 1995): 933–954.

U.S. House of Representatives, Committee on Ways and Means. *Overview of Entitlement Programs: 1992 Greenbook*. Washington, DC: Government Printing Office, 1992.

Walsh, Mary. *"Doctors Wanted: No Women Need Apply": Sexual Barriers in the Medical Profession, 1835–1975*. New Haven, CT: Yale University Press, 1977.

White, Joseph. "The Horses and the Jumps: Comments on the Health Care Reform Steeplechase," *Journal of Health Politics, Policy and Law* 20 (#2, summer 1995): 373–383.

White House Domestic Policy Council. *The President's Health Security Plan: The Complete Draft and Final Reports of the White House Domestic Policy Council*. New York: Times Books/Random House, Inc., 1993.

Witte, Edwin. *The Development of the Social Security Act*. Madison: University of Wisconsin Press, 1963.

Index

About the Author

GREG M. SHAW is associate professor of political science at Illinois Wesleyan University, where he teaches courses on American social policy and public opinion. He has written widely in these areas. His previous book, *The Welfare Debate* (2007), is also part of Greenwood/ABC-CLIO's Historical Guides to Controversial Issues in America series.